MANAGEMENT OF THE FRAIL ELDERLY
BY THE HEALTH CARE TEAM

Management of the Frail Elderly by the Health Care Team

by

JOHN R. WALSH, M.D.
Professor of Medicine
Head, Division of Gerontology
Oregon Health Sciences University
Chief, Section of Geriatric Medicine
Portland Veterans Administration Medical Center

RUTH ANN W. TSUKUDA, R.N., M.P.H.
Coordinator of Interdisciplinary Team Training in Geriatrics
Portland Veterans Administration Medical Center
Assistant Professor, School of Medicine
Oregon Health Sciences University

JUDY MILLER, R.N. M.S.N.
Assistant Professor, Department of Adult Health and Illness Nursing
School of Nursing
Oregon Health Sciences University

WARREN H. GREEN, INC.
St. Louis, Missouri U.S.A.

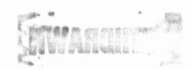

362
.19897
W225m

Published by

WARREN H. GREEN, INC.
8356 Olive Boulevard
St. Louis, Missouri 63132, U.S.A.

© 1989 by WARREN H. GREEN, INC.

ISBN No. 87527-349-1

Printed in the United States of America

PREFACE

This book about problems of the frail elderly is intended for health care providers in hospitals, nursing homes, residential and home health care. In these settings health care providers often encounter frustrations in dispensing care for the frail elderly who have multiple medical, mental and social problems. We have selected information on common disorders that hopefully will be helpful to health care providers. This book is not intended to be complete but summarizes some current issues and concerns about patient management.

Much of the material has been gathered from our experience teaching students who are collaborating in an interdisciplinary team teaching geriatric program. It is our belief that there is a body of knowledge about aging and the common problems of the frail elderly about which all disciplines should be conversant if we are to deliver better management to patients. Health care providers tend to gain more satisfaction working within areas of their own expertise and are understandably more comfortable in areas in which they are more knowledgeable. We often neglect areas in which we are unsure and, therefore, it is not surprising that physicians are inattentive to social problems and conversely that a social worker, for example, may not put medical problems in proper focus. In the extreme a denial of problems outside of one's area of competence tends to polarize concepts into strictly medical or social models. Obviously, older people may have problems at either end of the spectrum. However, the frail elderly so often have varying combinations of problems that require knowledge from many disciplines. Each discipline interacting in a team management concept should have a working knowledge of disorders outside of their own area of expertise which may influence their recommendations. Therefore, our goal is to provide a reasoned scientific basis for management, built on an understanding of the aging process and its influence on functional ability of the aged person.

An effective team approach to the composite needs of the frail elderly depends largely on competent joint assessment, and a willingness to exchange information to formulate and deliver an effective treatment plan. The size of the team is dependent on the resources and environments. A team may include only a physician, nurse and social worker or may be composed of representatives of a variety of disciplines such as: physician, nurse, social worker, pharmacist, dietician, speech, occupational, recreational, correctional and physical therapists, psychologist, psychiatrist, dentist, physician assistant, nurse practitioner, audiologist, optometrist and others depending on the nature of the underlying disorder. The size, notwithstanding, health care providers must assume responsibility for this segment of society since many of the disorders mentioned in this book are treatable even if present in a climate of underlying chronic disease.

Focal points of this book are the significance of functional and mental status assessment for more suitable placement of elderly patients, the compelling problems of urinary incontinence, overmedication, and immobility, and the rapid surfacing of ethical issues. Furthermore, it is our hope that health care providers will develop skills in anticipating and preventing complications that predictably hasten downhill progression, institutionalization, and ultimately death. An essential element in management is thoughtful evaluation and intervention yet, utilizing good judgment to avoid risks of drugs and procedures, coupled with an appropriate recognition of limitations of intervention, the aggregate of which is to encourage self–sufficiency in the elderly. Conversely, the hazards of inappropriate therapy are emphasized. The reader will obviously recognize that there are abundant unanswered questions and that the answers to dilemmas about who should receive care, and the quality and quantity of such care are just a few of the socioeconomic, medical, mental and ethical issues and controversies that need further exploration.

John R. Walsh, M.D.
Ruth Ann W. Tsukuda, R.N., M.P.H.
Judy Miller, R.N., M.S.N.

CONTENTS

MANAGEMENT OF THE FRAIL ELDERLY BY THE HEALTH CARE TEAM

Part 1
AGING IN AMERICA

CHAPTER 1

OVERVIEW OF AGING

LIFE SPAN, LIFE EXPECTANCY

The socioeconomic, medical, and psychological problems of growing old warrants not only concern but a mobilization of resources to address the evolving problems. Currently in the United States, there are 23 million people over age 65. It is estimated that by the year 2030, when the peak of the post World War II baby boom will be reaching 65, the United States will have more than 50 million elderly, or approximately twice the present number. But even more significant is the staggering increase in the number of persons over 75 years of age, the frail elderly, a segment of the aged that will have the greatest impact on the health care system. While seemingly incredulous, the older population itself is aging. By the year 2000, more than one-half of the over 65 year age group will be above 75 years of age, and by 2040 there will be eight million people over 80 years of age, about three times the number that existed in 1980. The rapid growth of the frail elderly will impose an extra burden on all levels of health care but especially on home health and nursing home care. Fifteen percent of those over 75 years of age are home-bound and 5% of those beyond age 65 are in nursing homes. There are presently 1.3 million people residing in nursing homes with 95% over age 65. Seventy-five percent of nursing home residents are greater than 75 years old. Of the over 85-year-old group, 21.6% are currently residing in nursing homes. The average age of residents in nursing homes is 82 years.

Many factors increase the risk of nursing home placement such as absence of a spouse, recent hospital discharge, incontinence, confusion or dementia. The typical nursing home resident is female, white, and widowed. With the increasing numbers of people reaching older age, it is estimated that about 20% of all elderly will eventually reside in a nursing home before dying. The dramatic anticipated increase in both absolute and relative propor-

4

tions of older people introduces the question of changing values of the younger members of our society as they face support of a rapidly increasing number of less productive old people. For example; will rigid criteria be established for care of the elderly or will there even be denial of care, with the elderly themselves assuming responsibility for their own care; will early retirement be interdicted and will retirement age be further extended?

A distinction must be made between life span and life extectancy. Human life span is finite for the species. For man the maximal life span is 115 years. Reports of people living past this age have raised suspicion of methods used in calculating birth dates. Life expectancy in the United States (average length of life) had increased from approximately 47 years in the year 1900 to 74 years today. The average life expectancy for white women is 78 years and for white men 70 years. With the decline in the number of infant deaths, control of infectious diseases and improvement in living conditions, diet, and sanitation, more people are living to an older age. Chronic disease has superceded acute disease in the aging population so that today's challenge is to prevent, or if impossible, to manage disability to make life more livable.

Society today is preoccupied with improving the environment and introducing healthy lifestyles as a means to prepare for a healthy problem-free old age. Appropriate exercise such as walking, jogging, weight reducing diets, interdiction of cigarette smoking and alcohol are enthusiastically embraced as a means to postpone chronic diseases such as stroke, coronary artery disease, cancer, diabetes, arthritis, emphysema, and liver cirrhosis. Already there has been a decline in deaths from cardiovascular disease and stroke attributed but not conclusively shown to be due to better lifestyle and treatment of hypertension. But workers in the field of aging have differing concepts and often interpret data differently. On the one hand, it has been suggested that a consequence of improving lifestyle will eventually result in the mean age of death approaching 85 years instead of the present 74 years, and that needs for medical care in later life will decrease (1). On the other hand, a contradictory viewpoint suggests that evidence supports a rapidly increasing number of old people who will experience a longer period of diminishing vigor beset by chronic disease for a larger proportion of their lifetime, therefore, medical care needs are likely to increase substantially (2-5).

A greater number of frail elderly people with chronic diseases, the projected need for more prostate and cataract operations and hip replacements (3), need for nursing home placement or other alternative forms of care, the increasing incidence of dementia, falls, and incontinence in this population would support a forecast for expanded health care needs unless solutions are forthcoming to prevent these problems or manage them more effectively. Presently preventive strategies with the goal to post-pone the onset of some chronic disease seems reasonable. Health care professionals must educate people about the benefits of a healthy lifestyle and the responsibility that each individual has to themselves and to society for being accountable for their own self-care. On the other hand, we must expect that with advanced age the frail elderly will still be beset by multiple disorders derived from the biological decline of old age and the diseases specific to old age. The most serious concomitant of chronic disease is func-tional disability with its resultant dependency requiring increas-ing care and support. Meeting these dependency needs is a chal-lenge to our health delivery system and research is needed to prevent chronic disease or manage it more effectively.

The manner in which health care professionals view aging greatly influences the outcome of health care services. A negative point of view that aging is a stage of dying will marshall minimal efforts to aid the elderly. On the other hand, a positive recogni-tion that small increments of improvement can be obtained by even partial correction of problems will minimize disability and promote better acceptance of self-care. This latter concept must be enthusiastically endorsed if interdisciplinary team management is to be successful. Management of the frail elderly, however, must be realistic with recognition of limitations to overly aggressive treatments that are harmful to this frail population. Nevertheless, good judgment must be exercised so as not to deny therapy that may be helpful. These decisions are not easily made and require considerable experience and thorough consideration of each patient.

HUMANE TREATMENT

For some health care professionals, care of the frail elderly is often not considered a rewarding experience, the thrill of cure is absent, and increments of improvement are slow with almost imperceptible change over long periods of time. Even cure of acute episodes of illness superimposed on underlying chronic disease fails to evoke enthusiasm because it is viewed as an episodic event in a climate of overwhelming disability. The patient is still on a gradual, albeit variable, downhill course from underlying chronic disorders. Yet, the quality of the patient's life is frequently influenced by the alleviation of an acute episode of illness, a minor alteration in the environment or the partial improvement of functional ability from a chronic disorder.

In contrast to the health provider's expectations, some frail old people with chronic ailments have fewer expectations of life and usually do not look for miraculous cures. They are most appreciative of time and interest shown them and grateful for small increments of improvement. On the other hand, if the patient and their health care providers routinely resign themselves to their disabilities, a feeling of hopelessness and insufficient support will prevail, and predictable premature incapacitation will ensue.

While health professionals must be realistic and recognize their limitations in treating the frail elderly patient, too often there is a prevailing attitude that life is almost over, therefore, it is a kindness to withhold treatment. Osler's aphorism "pneumonia is a friend of the elderly" is applicable to terminal stages of illness but it becomes a questionable concept when globally applied to all frail elderly people. Rehabilitative measures and appropriately aggressive therapy have been beneficial for many frail old people today. An example albeit a selected one is a recent study of medical intensive care for elderly patients which indicates that although hospital mortality was higher for older patients (16% for those over 75 years old, 14% for the 65-74 year old group and 8% for the 55-64 year old group) and mortality one year after hospital discharge was 44% for those older than 75 years, over 90% of those alive after one year were living at home (6). On the other hand, some invasive diagnostic and surgical procedures in frail old people are harmful and therefore should be undertaken only if the results will lead to a beneficial decision about the care of the patient. Unquestionably the establishment of criteria or guidelines for making such decisions will accrue with evaluation of our experience and through dialogue concerning treatment by all interested disciplines. In these determinations there is no justification for judgments based on the perceived social worth of people predicated on diminished or finite resources and the increasing needs of larger numbers of frail elderly people. Individual needs must not necessarily be subordinated to social needs.

There is no guarantee that whatever resources are saved will be used for any better purpose (7). Obviously, there are some elderly people and their families who have unrealistic expectations of the health care system. In these circumstances where the patient, his family and health providers disagree it is important that the health care team set realistic goals that are clearly understood by the patient and family.

THE GERIATRIC PATIENT

There are several aphorisms or guidelines (Table 1.1) that all health care professionals should be acquainted with when caring for the elderly. Many frail elderly (over 75 years old) are in good health even though they have less physiological reserve capacity. While young and middle age adults are usually healthy, illnesses suffered by them are usually episodic, single acute diseases. However, as people age they accumulate problems and become the greatest consumers of health resources. Moreover, there is much undiscovered disease found through screening examinations of the elderly (8), some of which interferes with functional activity but, nonetheless, often treatable. Diabetes, cardiac disease, anemia, depression, incontinence, and disorders causing falls are super-

---

TABLE 1.1
AGING MAXIMS

- Aging is not synonymous with illness
- Most elderly are in good health
- Aging decreases physiological reserve capacity
- Illness/disability incorrectly perceived as aging
- Elderly minimize problems, reluctant to report illness
- Frail elderly acquire multiple physical, mental and social problems
- Multiple problems require multiple drugs, with high risk of side effects
- Conspicuous incidence of dementia, depression, incontinence and falls
- Characterized by multiple losses: vision, hearing, income, friends, health, social supports, etc.
- Atypical clinical presentation of disease
- Increased severity and slower recovery from acute illness

imposed on declining physiological reserve capacity, the aggregate of which interferes with ability to adequately function. The older one gets, the more evident the decline (Figure 1.1), the only variable being the rate of decline. It is reasonable to assume that a point will be reached at which function will be insufficient to sustain life.

Many old people learn to come to terms with physiological limitations and often transcend incapacities especially if they have adequate support systems. The frail elderly, however, have substantial decrements in physical and mental function as well as reduced socioeconomic and support system capabilities, factors which determine placement (Figure 1.2). They are, therefore, more vulnerable to disease, accidents, and risk of complications from drugs, diagnostic and therapeutic procedures, surgery and institutionalization. There is slower recovery after infections, surgical procedures and drug reactions, and more profound symptoms are observed with anemia, hyponatremia, dehydration and infections as compared to younger adults. The greater the biological

Biological Decline of Aging

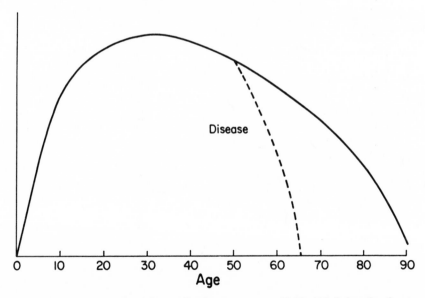

Figure 1.1. An incremental growth phase occurs until the third decade; thereafter physiological function progressively declines. Disease hastens the downhill progression.

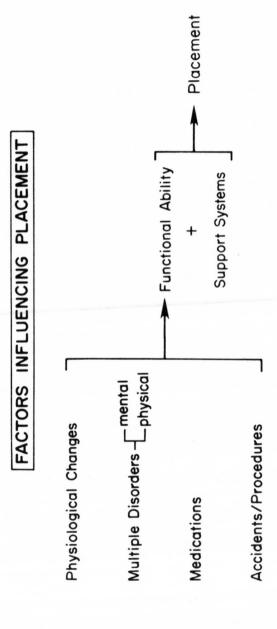

Figure 1.2. Interaction of physical, mental and socioeconomic factors that determine degree of dependency, e.g., living at home, congregate housing, room and board facility, or a nursing home.

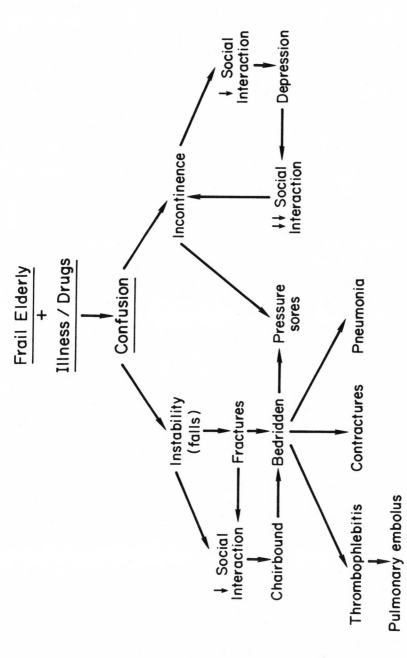

Figure 1.3. Sequence of events in frail elderly patients. Predictable patterns allow anticipation of each successive complication. The goal is to prevent each subsequent downward step.

decline, the more likely that these insults may start an inexorable downhill course resulting in institutionalization or death.

Differentiating functional losses related to the normal aging process from chronic degenerative disease is a dilemma. Many doctors, elderly patients themselves and their families mistakenly attribute illness and disability to aging changes. "It's old age, what else can you expect" implies that little can be done and has an accompanying fatalistic prognosis. Health care professions can circumvent this attitude by timely management of functional deficits rather than ascribing incapacity to old age.

Anticipatory Approach to Management

Multiple interacting disorders produce disability that is more than just additive in frail elderly patients. One diagnosis which explains problems so relevant to younger patients most often does not apply to the elderly (9). The older the person the more apt they are to have several problems. The resultant disabling functional loss often makes it difficult and sometimes impossible to cope with activities of daily living. For instance, an 80–year–old may function adequately in the community despite disabilities from a previous stroke, diminished vision, loss of hearing, disability from joint disease and frequency of urination from bladder outlet obstruction until a superimposed anemia or infection (urinary tract infection or pneumonia) produces confusion and episodes of falling or an adverse drug reaction tips the balance in favor of institutionalization. Even a mild illness in collaboration with multiple physical and mental problems often triggers a veritable cascade of complications (Figure 1.3) in frail elderly people. Disease in one organ system or the use of medications may accentuate other existing abnormalities creating and inexorable decremental course leading to incapacitation, dependency, institutionalization and eventually, death (10). In addition, hospitalized frail elderly paitents are exposed to predictable risks such as night time confusion (sundowning), falls, fractures, urinary incontinence, pressure sores, fecal impaction, adverse effects of drugs and procedures, and hazards of bed rest.

A major way to help most frail older people is to employ an anticipatory approach to prevent subsequent events that predictably trigger the downhill progression (Figure 1.3). An interdisciplinary team that utilizes anticipatory strategies will achieve success in forestalling institutional placement of frail elderly. The term "anticipatory medicine" describes an action–oriented prospective approach to management and is as much a part of preventive medicine as the promulgation of healthy life–style and behavioral strategies to prevent or postpone diseases such as atherosclerosis, lung cancer, emphysema and liver cirrhosis. It is particularly applicable to the frail elderly.

Multiple diseases often necessitate the use of multiple drugs which, are often responsible for adverse reactions. Drugs may cause confusion, incontinence and falls among other complications common to the elderly. Elderly persons have physical, mental and social problems which may occur independently or coexist interdependently in varying degrees. Older people have many losses including children, spouse, friends, work, vision, hearing, mobility to name a few. Because of so many losses it is particularly difficult to separate appropriate sadness from depression. Depression, a common disorder in this age group, may present nonspecifically. It may affect mood, cognitive function and physical state. Sixty percent have physical complaints (gastrointentinal dysfunction, intensified arthritic pain, etc.), 10% of patients thought to have dementia turn out to have depression. Somatic complaints of anorexia or weight change, sleep change, loss of energy, psychomotor retardation (slowing of speech, thinking, movement), agitation, and severe or intractable pain are frequently observed in varying degrees. Older people are less apt to attempt suicide but are more successful because of greater intent. Some patients develop a sick or dependent role and underrate their potential abilities. This negative attitude accentuates their incapacity and tends to delay or prevent rehabilitation. A physician alone cannot effectively deal with all the multiple physical, mental and socioeconomic problems of patients and their families. Health care has become too complicated to be an unshared responsibility. The use of an interdisciplinary approach to care is a solution to this dilemma.

Functional Capacity

Health care professionals, in addition to being concerned about integrating clinical signs and symptoms, laboratory and x-ray results to arrive at a medical diagnosis must collect data about the patient's capacity to function in his/her environment and ascertain the limitations that may be imposed by any physical impairment, abnormal psychological state, and deficits in social support before making recommendations that often will alter a patient's life-style. The health care team must assess what the patient can and will do when disabled by a stroke, arthritis, dementia, Parkinson's disease and other incapacitating illnesses. The health care team must measure abilities associated with self-care in addition to making specific diagnoses and writing drug prescriptions. A costly diagnostic work-up may be of questionable benefit if little or no attention is given to the patient's environment, support systems, or lack of resources that may make it impossible to follow instructions or participate in self-care. Health care professionals often do not pay attention to functional effects of physical or mental impairments with a goal to maximize the ability of patients to function in their environment. Basic activities of daily living (ADL) that keep an individual fed, clothed, toileted and clean and instrumental activities of daily living including cooking, cleaning, laundering, use of telephone, transportation, managing money or taking medicines are important factors that contribute to independent living or if deficient may lead to placement (Figure 1.2).

Unusual Presentation of Disease

Disease often presents in a vague and unclassical way in the elderly (11). Classical symptoms are replaced by nonspecific ones, most commonly, refusal to eat or drink, weight loss, disinterest in surroundings, withdrawal from activities, falling, incontinence, confusion, and worsening dementia. Older people have a blunted response to pain and a heart attack (myocardial infarction) may occur without pain. Painless myocardial infarction occurs in 20 to 80% of patients over age 65 (12, 13). Shortness of breath may replace the typical chest pain (angina pectoris) of an anginal attack and is called an anginal equivalent. Weakness and confusion from congestive heart failure may obscure angina. Dyspnea may occur after meals or at night. An acute abdomen may be heralded by confusion or loss of appetite rather than pain. Fever may be minimal or absent, the white blood cell count normal or only slightly elevated and abdominal tenderness inconspicuous in some elderly people with appendicitis, cholecystitis, diverticulitis and intraabdominal abscess (14). Pneumonia may lack physical signs of fever, leukocytosis and cough (15). Bacteremia (bacteria in blood stream) may not cause fever in elderly people (16). Malignant disease may be silent with the unexpected finding of a mass without clinical symptoms or the occurence of a fever of unknown origin. Depression may accentuate medical problems such as arthritis rather than appearing as sadness.

Thyrotoxicosis (hyperthyroidism), an overactive functioning thyroid gland, in elderly people may be clinically different than in younger adults (17). The hypermetabolic symptoms of nervousness, sweating, ravenous appetite with loss of weight, frequent stools, may be absent and the pulse may not be rapid. The thyroid gland may not be enlarged (absence of a goiter) in up to 40% of patients; atrial fibrillation frequently the only overt sign, often suggests a heart problem, and loss of appetite, weight loss and constipation which are atypical findings of thyrotoxicosis tends to direct attention to a colonic cancer. Apathetic thyrotoxicosis is a term applied to a hyperthyroid patient usually elderly, and who presents with weight loss, muscle wasting, lethargy, failure to thrive and depression. Thyroid function should be assessed in every older patient with a recent onset of atrial fibrillation, unexplained congestive heart failure, or unexplained worsening of angina pectoris.

Hypothyroidism is difficult to diagnose in a frail elderly person. Slow cerebration, lethargy, cold intolerance, constipation, poor hearing, thinning of the outer one–third of the eyebrows and dry skin are typical findings of hypothyroidism but may be found in normal frail elderly people in the absence of thyroid hormone deficiency. If the skin and hair are coarse, the voice hoarse and there is "gelling of the reflexes" (slow relaxation), the clinical diagnosis is more secure. However, these findings may be absent in hypothyroidism of elderly people. Hypothyroidism should always be considered in a patient with either dementia or hypothermia.

Clinical features of a disorder may be tempered or even masked by a change in life style or by concomitant disease. Limitation of activity by arthritis or weakness may conceal angina pectoris (chest pain) because with less activity there is diminished oxygen myocardial (heart muscle) demand and therefore angina is not provoked. Peripheral vascular disease or COPD which restrict walking or other activity may conceal angina pectoris. Similarly, a patient with angina pectoris may be relieved of symptoms if he becomes sedentary because of a stroke. Another example is the patient with peripheral vascular disease whose leg pains which result from insufficient blood oxygen supply during walking may have less leg pain when shortness of breath from another disorder restrict walking. On the other hand, a superimposed disease may worsen another disability, for example, residual weakness of a left leg from a stroke may place greater stress on an arthritic right hip and knee. Similarly treatment of the incapacity from Parkinson's disease in a patient who also has severe dementia may impose additional stress on the family because of excessive wandering. Many other clinical variations of modification of clinical features in the aged will be seen throughout the progress of this book.

Senility (Failure to Thrive)

The term senility, a global term that implies a progressive loss of physical and mental function is meaningless (11, 18). To some senility is synonymous with dementia, to others it connotes "failure to thrive" a term suggesting dwindling function in an elderly person. The term "dwindles" has also expressed this progressive deterioration. These terms imply that age itself is responsible and reflects a denial that intervention can change the outcome, thereby fostering a negative attitude that dampens any search for remedial or even partially correctible causes. Atypical and non-specific clinical presentation of disease in the frail elderly fits the obscure "failure to thrive" constellation of findings. Weakness, fatigue, loss of appetite, loss of interest, falls, immobility, and mild confusion are common complaints often ascribed to senility or "failure to thrive" which clearly demand assessment. The underlying diagnosis inevitably will be missed if the patient is not appropriately assessed.

INTERDISCIPLINARY COLLABORATION

Obviously no single discipline or physician can handle the complex interrelated health care needs of the elderly. The unique skills and knowledge of a social worker, dietician, pharmacist, psychologist, physical and occupational therapists, audiologist, optometrist, dentist and other health professionals may be needed in addition to the physician and the nurse (Figure 1.4). Essentially the objectives of providing health care services are to enhance functioning capabilities, to match services to needs, to simplify regimens (drugs, activities of daily living, etc), and to reduce inappropriate utilization of hospital and/or nursing home facilities. Each discipline provides assessment and management skills to develop comprehensive treatment plans and to facilitate rehabilitation programs. Although team members work independently, as

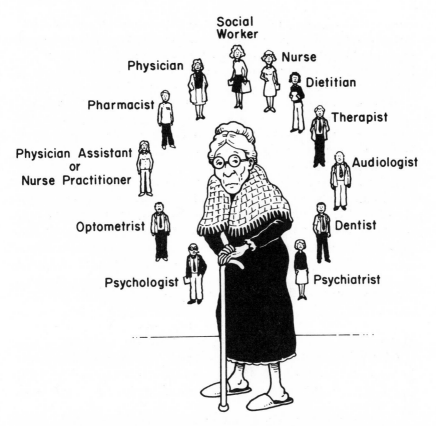

Figure 1.4. Focus of the interdisciplinary team is the elderly patient.

well as interdependently, the cornerstone of teamwork is a sharing of planning and action with a joint responsibility for outcomes. The knowledge base of the team is increased through the exchange of information, joint assessment and a collaborative definition of a treatment plan. The interdisciplinary approach requires frequent interaction among team members. To be effective the interdisciplinary team must be action-oriented with a commitment to accept responsibility for expediting management in their respective area of expertise. The process is both an educational and service-oriented experience.

Members of the interdisciplinary team must learn to work together, must have respect for each other's skills and knowledge, must be open to new concepts and willing to share valuable experience and expertise. Expectations of how the team will work must be clearly outlined, goals and tasks must be spelled out. Team members who glibly outline tasks for others, but are unwilling to participate or arrange for patient management in their own discipline, create poor morale and sometimes evoke hostility of other team members, the result of which is reflected in poor care. Conference discussion should not inordinately outweigh participation in patient care. In addition to their own direct patient care activities, team members should have the ability to listen, to trust, to be open and to communicate clearly and effectively, and have a willingness to cooperate with others in providing health care services. In the decision making process the team must set short and long range goals for management of patients. Patient issues must be outlined and thoroughly discussed by team members. The decision of who does what and when must be addressed if the goals of team work are to be accomplished.

STEREOTYPIC DEVALUATION OF THE OLD

In a society fraught with misconceptions and stereotypes, it should come as no surprise that the elderly are often the objects of false beliefs, biases, and discriminatory processes. These biases thrive in an atmosphere devoid of facts. In 1975, Dr. Robert Butler coined the term "ageism" to describe these practices. He states:

> "Ageism can be seen as a process of systematic stereotyping of and discrimination against people because they are old, just as racism and sexism accomplish this with skin color and gender. Old people are categorized as senile, rigid in thought and manner, old-fashioned in morality and skills. . . Ageism allows the younger generation to see older people as different from themselves; thus, they subtly cease to identify with their elders as human beings" (19).

Although familiar to all of us, the impact of ageism becomes more dramatic if described even more specifically. The elderly are often viewed as being pretty much alike, a homogeneous group of people who have ceased to be productive, functional, or creative members of society. There seems to be some mythical age where activity and attractiveness decline, intellectual capacity diminishes, sexuality ends, physical activity decreases, and health declines. These beliefs are reinforced by a society which bombards us through a media which shows old people to be foolish, senile, lecherous, feeble, helpless, deaf, and constipated. In contrast, we are exposed to images that define attractiveness and successfulness as being young, slim, intelligent, physically attractive, and productive. Health professionals often share these same myths and stereotypes and frequently reinforce society's negative attitude.

Perhaps even more important than the concept of "ageism," itself, are its consequences as these prejudices are acted out in society. In *Why Survive? Being Old in America*, Butler describes some of these consequences:

— Societal and political policies that discriminate against the elderly
— Disdain or dislike for the elderly
— Avoidance of the elderly
— Discriminatory practices in housing, employment and services of all kinds
— Protection of younger individuals against their own fears of growing old or ill, and of death itself
— Assumption by some elderly that the myths are true, resulting in decreased self-esteem, satisfaction, and productivity (19).

Thus, it is obvious that attitudes toward the elderly influence their quality of life. Attitudes are comprised of three parts: knowledge or cognition, affect or feeling, and action (20). The feelings health professionals have toward older persons and toward the aging process itself directly affect how we interact with members of this large segment of the population. If we fear our own aging process or dislike working with people whose illnesses are unlikely to be "cured," it will affect our interaction processes (21). What we know and think about aging also affects how we treat elders. In the chapters that follow, aging, health, and illness will be discussed in depth. However, an understanding of the source and extent of negative attitudes increases awareness regarding our own beliefs and how these beliefs may influence our practice.

Most research concludes that attitudes toward the elderly vary among different cultures and that these attitudes also vary at different times. It does seem that as life expectancy has lengthened and as society has become more industrialized and more technological, attitudes toward the elderly have become more negative (22).

Attitudes toward aging and the aged have been the focus of many research endeavors over the past years. The following conclusions regarding attitudes are widely accepted:

1. Most people have mixed feelings about aging, rating old
   age positive on some dimensions and negative on others.
2. More stereotypes are associated with old age than other
   ages.
3. A majority of persons both young and old hold many
   stereotypes toward aging (22).

Once again, it seems that the common belief is that to be
young is good and becoming old is bad.

The effect that ageism has can be generalized in many ways.
It is not unusual for younger persons to feel pity toward the
elderly. The lives of the elderly seem not to be worth living. The
elderly seem to be out of pace with the rest of the younger members of society. They are unproductive. How differently the young
perceive themselves and society. It almost seems impossible for
some young people to think of themselves as becoming old, or to
describe how they see themselves at 80. Therefore, the lives of the
elderly are not perceived to be similar to their own. Old age is not
viewed as a natural stage of life with its own achievements, and
philosophies, acquired through accumulated experience. The
values of today's society tend towards independence and productivity, not wisdom as was valued in the past. Rapid technological
turnover and the threat of obsolescence generates a fast–paced
life style where rapid decision–making and fast response to
demands for change are the norm. Aged persons who do not fit
into this societal mold may be ignored, isolated and may even
become the subject of ridicule or as discussed, they become the
subject of stereotyping.

One possible cause for a lack of understanding of the aged,
is the tendency for younger and older members of society to
be somewhat separated from each other. As our own society
has become more mobile, children have moved greater distances
away from their parents, and consequently the exposure to
aging family members has decreased. Another more recent
phenomenon has been the decision of large segments of the
elderly to move to adult retirement communities, thus choos-
ing to segregate themselves from younger generations. Often
this choise is based on such factors as climate, cost, convenience, and environmental planning which has addressed the specific housing and social needs of the aged. It is not usually an
attempt to purposefully segragate oneself from younger persons
and most of those residing in such communities maintain meaningful family relationships. Taken to its most disturbing extreme, this

age segregation can be seen in the numbers of old persons residing in institutional settings, sometimes inappropriately. Bromley states that this age segregation has resulted in fewer encounters with older persons, thus their contrast with "normal" human adults is even more marked. He concludes that segregation itself labels persons as discarded (23).

It is important to understand myths and stereotypes from the perspective of society, from the perspective of individuals, and also from an organizational perspective. Personal attitudes positive or negative, are evident in interaction patterns, while the attitude of society can foster either positive or negative actions. It can also be said that each organization through the manner in which it conducts its work, also influences the behavior of those who work within it. Organizations, particularly hospitals and nursing homes, assume the behavioral characteristics of its staff and develop an institutional personality. It is obvious to those who work in environments serving the elderly that some organizations are more able to foster a work climate which emphasizes positive attitudes toward aging.

Just as society and individuals must examine their value system as it relates to the aged, so must long term care centers, hospitals, home care agencies, and other organizations which care for the elderly. Debunking the myths and devaluing stereotypes which influence the way staff perceive the old and subsequently care for them is an on-going challenge. Negative attitudes limit caregivers in their provision of sensitive and respectful care (20). Furthermore, although knowledge itself is important toward increasing awareness of attitudes, it is no guarantee that behavioral changes will be observed in practice. Staff education is only one measure to help weaken the influence of negative attitudes. Other measures include such things as recognition of the rights of individuals to participate in decisions regarding their health care; recognition of the integrity of the individual as a complex bio-psycho-social being; and providing an environment which fosters the provision of high quality health care services by a staff which is not only technically knowledgeable, but also sensitive to individual patient needs and who show respect for the people they serve.

In conclusion, although myths and stereotypes of aging are still common, as our population continues to age and as the aged become a more vocal and powerful group in society, it can be expected that once again societal attitudes toward the aged will change. It is predictable that as the offspring of the baby boom eventually become the predominant older group the force of their numbers will ultimately shift emphasis of the market place to patronize this aging population and stereotypes will be changed.

REFERENCES

1. Fries, JF: Aging, natural death and the compression of morbidity. *N Engl J Med, 202:*130–135, 1980.

2. Siegel, JS: In *Proceedings of the Second Conference on the Epidemiology of Aging,* Haynes, SG and Feinlieb, M (Eds.). NIH Publication No. 80-969, Washington, DC, US Government Printing Office 1980, pp. 218–315.

3. Feinlieb, M: In *Proceedings of the Second Conference of the Epidemiology of Aging,* Haynes, SG and Feinlieb, M (Eds.). NIH Publication No. 80-969, Washington, DC, US Government Printing Office, 1980, p. 359.

4. Brody, JA: Life expectancy and the health of older persons. *J Am Geriatr Soc, 30:*681–683, 1982.

5. Schneider, EL; Brody, JA: Aging, natural death, and the compression of morbidity: Another view. *N Engl J Med, 309:*854–855, 1983.

6. Campion, EW; Mulley, AG; Goldstein, RL: Medical Intensive Care for the Elderly. A study of current use, costs and outcomes. *JAMA, 246:*2052, 1981.

7. Jonsen, AR; Siegler, M; Winslade, WJ: *Clinical Ethics: A Practical Approach to Ethical Decisions in Clinical Medicine.* New York: Mac Millan, 1982.

8. Williamson, J; Stokoe, IH; Gray, S, *et al.:* Old people at home: Their unreported needs. *Lancet, 1:*1117–1120, 1964.

9. Hodkinson, HM: Nonspecific presentation of illness. *Br Med J, 4:*94, 1973.

10. Irvine, PW: Patterns of Disease: The Challenge of Multiple Illness, In *Geriatric Medicine: Fundamentals of Geriatric Care,* Vol. II, Cassel and Walsh (Eds.). New York: Springer-Verlag, 1984, pp. 82–88.

11. Hodkinson, HM: *Common Symptoms of Disease in the Elderly.* 2nd edit. London: Blackwell, 1980.

12. Tinker, GM: Clinical Presentation of Myocardial Infarction in the Elderly. *Age Aging, 10:*237–240, 1981.

13. Harris, R: Cardiovascular Diseases in the Elderly. *Med Clin North Am, 67:*379, 1983.

14. Norman, D; Yoshikawa, TT: Intraabdominal Infections in the Elderly. *J Am Geriatr Soc, 31:*677, 1983.

15. Smith, IM: Infections in the elderly. *Hosp Pract, 17:*69–85, 1982.

16. Gleckman, RA; Roth, RM: Afebrile bacteremia in the elderly. *Intern Med for the Specialist, 5:*105, 1984.

17. Ryan, AJ; Davis, PJ: Unusual Clinical Manifestations of Hyperthyroidism in the Elderly. *Geriatr Med Today, 2:*49–54, 1983.

18. Comfort, A: *Practice of Geriatric Psychiatry.* New York: Elsevier, 1980.

19. Bulter, R: *Why Survive? Being Old in America.* New York: Harper and Row, 1975.

20. Miller Sr., P: Rx for the Aging Person: Attitudes. *J Gerontolo Nurs, 2(2):*22–26, 1976.

21. Adelson, R; Nasti, A; Sprafkin, JN; Marinelli, R; Premavera, LH; Gorman, BS: Behavioral Ratings of Health Professionals' Interactions with the Geriatric Patient. *Gerontologist, 22:*277–281, 1982.

22. Palmore, EB: Attitudes Toward the Aged. *Research on Aging 4(3):* 333–348, 1982.

23. Bromley, DB: Approaches to the Study of Personality Changes in Adult Life and Old Age, In *Studies in Geriatric Psychiatry*, Isaacs, AD and Post, F (Eds.). New York: Wiley, 1978.

CHAPTER 2

THE PROCESS OF AGING

BEYOND WRINKLES:
BIOLOGICAL CHANGES OF AGING

As people age many body functions show a progressive decline beginning about age 30 and persisting for the remainder of the life span, the only variable being the slope of the decline. With increasing age, there is a greater variability from one person to another. All organs do not suddenly reach a critical level of dysfunction producing total system failure at a designated time. Morphological and physiological changes affect organ systems to a different degree in each individual (1, 2). Therefore, some renal, cardiovascular, and pulmonary functions show a 50% decline between the ages of 30 and 80 while others exhibit smaller decreases. Some functions vary little throughout adult life such as electrolyte composition, pH values, or core temperature. However, if disturbed by disease or environmental factors recovery occurs at significantly slower rates in elderly persons.

Organs of the healthy aged are usually smaller than those of younger adults, a notable exception being the prostate gland. Atrophy is the general rule in old age, aging being characterized by a decrease in body cells. Cells become larger with age, therefore, the total body mass may not decrease despite a decrease in the number of cells. Mitotic cells are capable of many divisions, before dying. Cells of the skin or the intestinal tract for example are constantly replaced throughout life. Other cells such as nerve cells are postmitotic cells which must last a lifetime and cannot be replaced when they degenerate nor can they repair themselves when damaged. Therefore, there is a gradual degenerative process throughout the life span of an individual that is inevitable.

Body composition changes with age. Total body water of males decreases from about 62% to 53% partially due to an increase in body fat as muscle mass decreases (3). Extracellular water remains stable, but intracellular water decreases appreciably.

The increase in body fat often obscures other losses, although the distribution of fat in women is largely over the chest, waist, hips, and thighs, while in men is accumulates in the waist, lower abdomen, and chest. The sedentary habits of elderly people may contribute to excess fat and reduced muscle mass. A loss of fat, especially over the thighs, occurs in the frail elderly, especially in the eighth and ninth decades.

Stature and Posture

The older one gets the shorter one becomes. A shrinkage in height begins after age 50 amounting to 3 cm in males and 5 cm for females over a lifetime (4, 5). This is due to shortening of the vertebral column. The major change is shrinkage of the intervertebral discs and collapse of osteoporotic vertebrae. The long bones show less significant shortening. The old person, therefore, has a shortened trunk and comparatively long extremities. Kyphosis or forward bending of the thoracic vertebrae produces the "dowagers hump" which in turn causes the neck to be held in extension for vision above the ground. Kyphosis leads to an increased anterior–posterior diameter of the chest (barrel chest).

There is slight flexion of the knees and hips. The inability to completely extend the lower leg with failure to lock the knee joint on standing quickly fatigues the quadricep muscles. There is little or no flexion at the ankle. Slow, small shuffling steps are taken and the older person is unsteady and fearful of falling. Furthermore, the older person walks and turns the body as a unit (en bloc) which causes imbalance and instability of gait.

Muscle: Muscle fibers decrease at a rate of 3–5% per decade after age 30 years (6). Muscle strength and endurance progressively decreases with age. The decline in strength is 30 to 50% from ages 20 to 80. These changes are magnified by immobility, lack of exercise and poor nutrition. Sedentary older people show greater atrophy than active people. Clearly, prolonged inactivity such as bed rest is responsible for muscle atrophy, weakness and diminished endurance. Exercise and reconditioning will improve muscle function at all ages but the extent of improvement decreases with age. The conclusion is obvious, that a carefully planned program of exercise for older people can prevent physical deterioration and improve functional abilities. However, any program must consider the limitations imposed by any disability that may be present.

Nutritional Changes

Caloric intake decreases with age due to reduced basal caloric requirement and diminished physical activity (7). A major problem especially with the frail elderly is loss of appetite, weight, strength and easy fatiguability rather than an overweight problem. Social isolation, depression, illness, and drugs contribute to loss of appetite along with the diminished caloric intake of aging. Improving the appetite is often a most important factor in rehabilitation to a higher level of independence.

Food restriction has been effective in increasing longevity in rats albeit the mechanism is unknown (8). However, applying this approach to people especially in a clinical setting has been difficult and more experimental evidence in humans is needed before it can be endorsed as a life style. Food restriction in rats or mice in addition to prolonging life also delays onset of elevated serum cholesterol and triglyceride (9), retards the normal onset of immunosenescence, and reduces the incidence of cancer to mention a few examples (10). There is much yet to be learned about dietary restriction especially in humans. The elderly and their health care providers seemingly are caught in the crossfire between proponents for weight loss on the one hand, and those who advocate varying degrees of obesity on the other. Studies on rats showing that caloric restriction doubled their lifespan has been widely acclaimed by the "thin is in" advocates to promote a host of weight reduction diets, natural versus synthetic foods, and health food fads. On the other side of the coin, "fat is beautiful" enthusiasts are attempting to gain acceptance for their life style. Studies, however, show that extremes of thinness and obesity are associated with increased mortality. On the other hand, people with mild to moderate obesity have been shown to survive the longest. In the absence of clear guidelines it would appear logical to follow sound, proven nutritional practices especially with the frail elderly and avoid costly food fads evangelistically endorsed by overnight experts. Obviously a weight reduction program is justified for conditions of excess obesity that worsens a functional disability.

Plasma levels of cholesterol and triglycerides increase in middle age and are higher in men than women. With advancing old age these levels begin to decrease in men (11). However, in women, there is a "postmenopausal overshoot" in cholesterol levels, the increased values being attributed to reduced estrogen levels. After age 70, there is a decline in triglycerides and cholesterol in women (11). Elevated lipids are risk factors for cardio-vascular disease and there is a possibility that the elderly group with lower lipid levels are a select group of survivors. In younger adults elevated triglycerides and cholesterol especially low density lipoprotein (LDL) cholesterol levels are considered high risk factors for atherosclerotic complications. In the elderly, these factors are less significant and the health care team should not be preoccupied by the same dietary restrictions as with younger adults.

In old age, there is a progressive decline in carbohydrate metabolism. Previous standards for interpreting abnormal plasma glucose levels after a standard oral glucose ingestion suggested that 50% of people over age 60 had diabetes. It was obvious that many of these older people with age-related changes in carbohydrate metabolism were not diabetic. A new set of criteria for interpreting blood sugar levels has been adopted which has removed literally millions of older people from the diabetic category (12). A fasting plasma glucose value of 140 mg/dl or more is diabetic and a glucose tolerance test is not necessary. A plasma glucose level above 140 mg/dl two hours after oral ingestion of 75 grams of glucose, associated with a fasting level below that level should be designated "impaired glucose tolerance" and should not be labelled as diabetic.

Sensory Changes

Sensory changes can critically affect the relationship of a person with his environment. It can hinder everyday activities and lead to feelings of isolation. Inability to read the newspaper, watch television, use the telephone or listen to the radio constricts the environment of an older person. Sensory deprivation can predispose to depression, paranoia and hallucinations. It can lead to accidents. A misdiagnosis of dementia may stem from sensory losses, for instance, wrong responses to questions due to hearing impairment, inability to recognize persons or objects, poor orientation to time or place related to visual problems.

Vision

Vision changes as people age. Visual changes influence ability to perform daily activities, shop, go up or down stairs, operate appliances, read, watch television, etc. With advancing age less light reaches the retina because of smaller pupils, loss of lens transparency and increased lens thickness. Consequently, older people have difficulty functioning in areas with low light levels and need more illumination than young adults. They need better light for reading and may for example, have difficulty reading a menu in a dimly lit restaurant. With age the elasticity of the lens decreases and elderly people are unable to focus on near objects, that is, they are farsighted. This is a normal process of aging called presbyopia which can be corrected with plus–power lenses for reading or bifocals.

Color perception fades with advancing age. The lens becomes yellow with age and filters out light of short wave length such as violet and blue light. Reds, oranges and yellows are relatively unchanged and are easier to differentiate. This has practical implications with color coding of pills or using color to identify rooms in a nursing home.

Problems with glare, particularly troublesome for older people are due to light scattered by the cornea but opacities of the lens (cataracts) occurring with age are especially responsible for major scattering of light causing glare. Elimination or minimization of glare is helpful for the safety and comfort of an older person. Glare from sunlight on large windowpanes should be minimized and glossy polished surfaces, and waxed floors that reflect light should be eliminated. Sunglasses, hats with brims or bills reduce the glare source of reflected light in the summertime or in winter when snow is on the ground. Glare from white uniforms in nursing homes and hospitals distorts facial features and consequently may cause failure of patients to recognize their health providers. Nursing homes and hospitals must become better informed about the effects of glare on older patients.

Visual impairment and blindness has an increasing prevalence in the aged. By age 80, 30% have poor vision (less than 20/100). Over 50% of blind persons are over age 65. The major causes of blindness in later life are glaucoma, macular degeneration, senile cataract and diabetic retinopathy.

The fat cushion behind the eye globe atrophies and the eyes appear sunken. The eyelids become lax, thinner and may droop. The lower lid loosens and falls away from the globe. Insufficient tearing causes dryness of the eyes. An arcus senilus, a peripheral corneal fatty deposition is invariably present.

Hearing

Hearing loss is prevalent in the elderly. About 30% of elderly over age 65 have hearing impairments. The incidence of hearing loss is 48 to 90% of residents living in nursing homes. Loss of hearing of high frequency sounds, presbycusis, is a degenerative change due to aging, therefore, it is more difficult to hear women or children's voices. The functional result is a reduced ability to understand or discriminate speech. The patient will usually hear only parts of words since consonants are usually high frequency and vowels are a lower frequency. Speech may be heard faintly, sounds muffled and indistinct, those afflicted have more difficulty hearing in an environment where there is competing background noise or multiple competing conversations such as at social gatherings and restaurants, attempting to converse with background noise from home appliances, radio or television. Measures that substantially enhance the ability of the hearing-impaired person to improve communication are to eliminate background noise, face the person in a well-lit room to allow lip reading, speak slowly, use low tones and do not shout. Women especially must not speak loudly since this increases high frequency sounds.

Taste and Smell

Taste and smell sensations are less acute with advancing age. Foods taste bland and older people may begin to use more salt, spices and sugar. Unpleasant odors may not disturb older people. However, they are less aware of noxious gas fumes, or spoiled foods.

Aging Changes of the Nervous System

Brain weight begins to drop from the third decade so that by age 80 the decrease may reach slightly over 15%. The significance of the loss of brain weight is unclear and there are many older persons in their eighth and ninth decades who have no loss of intellectual function. CT scans have shown an increase in the size of the ventricles especially in the eighth and ninth decades (13). Cerebral atrophy is diagnosed by the CT scan even in elderly people with little or no cognitive loss. A variable number of neurons are lost in the brain by 80 to 90 years of age (14). A small number of neuritic placques and neurofibrillary tangles are found in aged normal brains.

Aging changes in the spinal cord show a 30 to 50% loss of anterior horn cells in the lumbrosacral area (15). Peripheral nerves show degenerative changes with advancing age. A progressive slowing of maximum nerve conduction velocities in distal lower extremities occurs with aging. Ankle jerk reflexes are diminished or lost, proprioceptive and vibratory sensations are decreased or lost in the feet. Motor and sensory nerve conduction decreases. Diminished function in the spinal cord and peripheral nerves are responsible for some loss of strength, agility and perhaps gait problems in the elderly.

Renal Changes with Age

Advancing age produces significant changes in kidney functions. There is a 20% reduction in weight of the kidneys, from 250g at age 40 to 200g at age 80 (16). There is a loss of approximately 30% of the glomeruli between ages 30 to 80 years. In addition, approximately 10% of the remaining glomeruli are sclerosed in the eighth decade. Renal blood flow is progressively reduced by advancing age. The major physiological change is a progressive decline in the glomerular filtration rate (GFR) (17). Creatinine clearance, a practical method to measure GFR shows a decrease from 140 ml per minute to 97 ml per minute between ages 30 to 80 years. The serum creatinine determination itself is not a good measure of kidney function in the elderly. The serum creatinine may be normal when the GFR is appreciably decreased in elderly people. Creatinine is derived from muscle and muscle mass in the elderly is lower. Therefore, there is no change in serum creatinine but there is an age–related reduction in creatinine clearance. Practically, serum creatinine values must be above 1.5 mg/dl to be considered abnormal in the older person.

Fluid and electrolyte disorders are common in the elderly and have their origin in diminished renal function. The aged kidney's response to sodium deficiency is sluggish (18). With a reduction in salt intake the aged patient's response to conserve sodium by reducing urinary sodium excretion requires a longer time; twice as long as young individuals (T/2 17 hours in young vs 31 hours in the elderly). This makes an older person more vulnerable to develop dehydration from loss of blood volume after vigorous salt restriction for hypertension or cardiac failure. An acute illness or addition of a diuretic in this setting magnifies the fluid and electrolyte imbalance. The ensuing disorientation with loss of thirst and poor salt intake further intensifies symptoms and worsens impaired cardiac, renal and mental function.

Hyponatremia (serum sodium ⟨ 135 mEg/L) a frequent event in the elderly should always be anticipated in any febrile illness, after surgical procedures, and with drugs that modify fluid and electrolytes such as diuretics or water retaining drugs such as chlorpropramide. Water excess (intoxication) due to water retention usually due to oversecretion of antidiuretic hormone (ADH) results in hyponatremia. This occurs with pneumonia, meningitis, stroke, subdural hematoma, and stress of anesthesia or surgery in the elderly. Lethargy, weakness, confusion, anorexia and muscle cramps from hyponatremia may be misdiagnosed as depression, dementia or malignancy. Severe hyponatremia (sodium ⟨ 110 mEq/L) may cause seizures or coma.

Liver Changes with Aging

Liver weight correlates with total body weight and both decrease after age 50. Blood flow to the liver declines with aging amounting to a 50% reduction in advanced old age. Liver blood flow is a major determinant of liver clearance of some drugs such as propranolol and lidocaine (19). The liver is the principal site for enzymatic modification of drugs, some of which are modified by age. Oxidative pathways particularly hydroxylation and N-dealkylation are impaired in the elderly thereby reducing drug clearance from the liver and causing higher blood plasma concentrations. Therefore, the frail elderly population has a decreased ability to metabolize drugs.

Respiratory Function

Aging is associated with a gradual decline of pulmonary function. Vital capacity and forced expiratory volume in one second (FEV_1) decrease. With age there is an increase in alveolar–arterial oxygen difference due to a decrease of the arterial oxygen pressure (PaO_2) which may be partly caused by a decrease of oxygen diffusion from the alveoli to the blood or a mismatch of ventilation and perfusion. On the other hand, residual volume and functional residual capacity slowly increase with age.

Cardiovascular Changes with Age

With advanced age the wall of the aorta is thickened, elasticity is reduced, it becomes elongated and tortuous. With aortic stiffness the left ventricle must pump against increased impedence. The systolic blood pressure typically increases with age. Former beliefs that the elderly tolerate high blood pressure better than the young and that it is, therefore, a benign condition in old age, that old people need higher pressures to perfuse aging organs, that it is better tolerated in elderly women and that treatment of hypertension is too risky in the aged are unsupported by recent evidence.

Hypertension in the elderly is of two types: The typical elevated diastolic pressure which is practically always accompanied by an increased systolic pressure, and isolated systolic hypertension. The risk of stroke, congestive heart failure and myocardial infarction increases with age in hypertensive patients. Elderly hypertensives may be at greater risk to develop dementia of multi-infarct type, abdominal aneurysm and perhaps peripheral vascular insufficiency. In the elderly, systolic hypertension is a greater risk factor than diastolic pressure, especially at levels above 160 mm Hg. It has been suggested that systolic blood pressure above 180 mm Hg should be treated. However, if angina, congestive heart failure or transient ischemic attacks are present even in a patient with a systolic pressure of 160 mm Hg, treatment would be indicated.

The resting heart is virtually unchanged by aging. Although controversial there may be less output of blood from the heart under the stress of exercise. The older person cannot increase the heart rate as much as younger counterparts. Systolic blood pressure is higher after exercise and takes longer to return to the pre-exercise level in older individuals. During maximal prolonged exercise the cardiovascular system supports this activity by taking up and distributing oxygen to the working muscles. A measure of this aerobic ability is the maximal oxygen consumption (VO_2 max). VO_2 max is generally accepted as a measure of cardiorespiratory fitness. After a 2–5 minute exhausting treadmill run, VO_2 declines with advancing age. The extent of this age–related decline is influenced by physical conditioning, smoking and obesity. VO_2 max decreases with as little as 3 weeks of bedrest in previously active individuals, reflecting a loss of cardiovascular fitness, conversely, it increases after physical training. Exercise, therefore, improves aerobic activity and active individuals have a greater maximal aerobic activity and greater functional reserve than sedentary individuals. Some of the decline in cardiovascular reserve may be due to a sedentary lifestyle of elderly people rather than the aging process itself.

Temperature

The febrile response to infection is sometimes impaired in older people. The absence of fever may hinder recognition of an infection and delay initiation of treatment. Instead of fever, pneumonia may exhibit confusion, loss of appetite and weight.

The autonomic nervous system controls vital functions such as blood pressure, temperature, gastrointestinal motility, urinary bladder function and respiration. Orthostatic hypotension and accidental hypothermia have been ascribed to dysfunction of the autonomic nervous system.

EMOTIONAL AND BEHAVIORAL ISSUES OF AGING

Still another myth which may cause misconceptions is the false belief that as people age they develop severe psychological and memory problems. The frail elderly have confronted a lifetime of stress, physical and mental insults which may reasonably be expected to become apparent during their declining years. The cumulative losses, bereavement and issues of death and dying are inevitable issues confronted in the daily life of the frail elderly. Health care providers must understand these problems to deal effectively with the frail elderly and to separate these issues from depression and dementia that are more often found in this age group.

Mental Processes and Aging

One of the common fears as people grow older is that they are becoming "senile" or demented because they are more forgetful. Contrary to popular belief, old age is not a time of universal decline in mental alertness or function. In fact, early research often falsely interpreted age as the determinant factor in intellectual ability rather than such variables as educational level or health status. Recent research has shown that little, if any, loss occurs in normal elderly individuals when intelligence is measured in terms of stored information (20). Verbal abilities remain unchanged in the aged and may even increase, especially in those who have shown high or average intellectual ability as measured by the Wechsler Adult Intelligence Scale (WAIS). However, educational level, not age, positively affects outcomes on the WAIS. It is believed that intelligence functions related to experience, information or vocabulary tend to improve into old age (21). These functions are sometimes referred to as crystallized intelligence.

However, other processes are negatively affected by age. Abstract thinking and problem solving, tend to reach a peak in young adulthood and then slowly decline in later years. Atchley states that the number of errors made in solving problems rises steadily with age (22).

Perhaps one of the best documented changes that occurs with increased age is the slowing of response time (23). A small proportion of this loss in speed is attributable to reduced peripheral nerve transmission but it is primarily related to more central physiological mechanisms. However, the slowing of response time does not affect cognition and individual differences in psychomotor speeds are great. It has been hypothesized that this slowing in response time may explain why older persons do not score as high as their younger counterparts on timed or time-limited tasks; however, allowing for additional time does not improve the scores on the WAIS (24). Thus, factors other than slowed response time contribute to differences in scores.

Perception is the ability to receive, register, process and respond to a stimulus. In other words, it is the way in which the individual reacts to the environment. There are many changes in sensory and perceptual abilities that occur as a result of aging which influence the behavior of the elderly person. In the aged, faulty perception of the environment may lead to seemingly inappropriate behavior (25).

It is often said that, "You can't teach an old dog new tricks;" however, this does not apply universally to the aged. Older people can learn, but it may take longer. Motivation is a strong factor that affects learning. "Frequently, older persons do perform better on tasks that are personally relevant to them in comparison to their relatively poor performance on meaningless tasks" (23). In general, long term memory is retained, but the ability to commit new information to memory decreases with age. Some other memory changes are: a decline in the ability to fully recall newly learned material; a decline in memory which requires the reorganization or manipulation of stored material; decline in the use of spontaneous memory strategies; and decreased ability to remember visually presented material in contrast to material which is presented auditorially (26). Elderly people have difficulty in transferring information from short-term memory to long-term memory so deficits occur at this juncture (25). Finally, remote memory (learned long ago) is least affected by age. In general, material learned when a person is 15-25 years of age is retained best throughout life (25).

Personality is the combination of factors, both biological and environmental, which together form the unique attributes or character of an individual. It is not true that individuals undergo major personality changes as they age. The stereotype that all old people are crotchety, gruff, or unhappy is unfounded. Personality traits tend to be continuous throughout the lifespan. Older people tend to show the same personality characteristics as they did when they were younger. However, people tend to become more introverted and preoccupied with themselves as they age. Some changeable personality characteristics relate to an older person's interpretation of his environment. Older people tend to become more conservative, they are more comfortable with the status quo and resist change, they become more cautious, and may exhibit greater rigidity. Anxiety is more common and often focuses on the adversities of old age (21).

To conclude, there is no typical pattern of change in aging. Psychological change in old people is complex and individualized. It should be emphasized that psychological change reflects only one dimension of an individual's health. Although several cognitive changes occur in conjunction with the aging process, alterations in mental processes often reflect an alteration in health status. Frequently a rapid decline in any sphere of psychological ability, may be one of the earliest signs of deterioration in physical well being.

Psychological Theories of Aging

Although the literature is replete with different theories of aging, only three major theories will be discussed. These theories are disengagement, activity and continuity theories. In general, they attempt to explain the interaction process which occurs between man and his environment.

The oldest theory is the Disengagement Theory, based on a belief that as people get older they withdraw from society. It was viewed as an adaptive process to aging whereby starting in late middle age there was a mutual process of withdrawal between the individual and society. The individual gradually withdraws from various roles in life and turns attention inward thus decreasing interactions with others. Reciprocally, society disengages with the aging individual so that its priorities center on the perpetuation of society (22). When the disengagement process is complete both the individual and society have redefined their relationships with one another (27). It assumes that the successful adjusted older person has withdrawn from much social interaction and many social roles. It implies that as the older person's physical capabilities decline, roles change, and the world in which they live changes, the universal response is to withdraw from the world rather than adjust to it.

Although once a popular explanation of the aging process, the disengagement theory has lost favor and is considered to be too simplistic to explain the complex interacting variables which affect an individual response to aging. Furthermore, it has been shown that although many older persons do withdraw from society, many others choose to remain actively engaged. Therefore, it is not a universal theory, nor can it explain the changing relationships between older individuals and a society which accepts many of them as contributing valuable members.

The controversy surrounding Disengagement Theory resulted in the postulation of two counter theories, activity and continuity. Proponents of the Activity Theory suggest that a healthy adaptation to aging is associated with the maintenance of activity. As aging progresses it becomes more difficult to maintain activity levels reached during younger years. The cornerstone of the Activity Theory is the concept of substitution. As one ages and roles change, one activity is substituted for another. It assumes that substitutes are available, the person has the physical reserves necessary to participate in the substitution and that a substitute is wanted. Although substitution is one way of coping with loss, it may be difficult to achieve, and as a theory it fails to explain why some people remain active and others disengage (3, 22).

Finally, the Continuity Theory views aging as a developmental process whereby the individual is constantly interacting with a social environment. It does not support one universal adaptive response but instead allows for a variety of patterns to be exhibited by individuals. Continuity Theory implies a consolidation of commitments and redistribution of available time and energy among remaining roles. Successful aging is in part dependent on the ability to cope with or adapt to environmental stress (22).

To date, no theory has adequately addressed the adaptation process of aging. Successful aging is dependent upon the ability to maintain an acceptable self-concept and to accommodate the changes that will inevitably be faced.

Aging: Adaptation to Change

Butler and Lewis in *Aging and Mental Health* state: "It is imperative that older people continue to develop and change in a flexible manner if health is to be promoted and maintained. Optimal growth and adaptation can occur all along the life cycle when the individual's strengths and potential are recognized, reinforced, and encouraged by the environment in which he lives" (28).

One of the crucial situations facing old persons is adaptation to loss. Loss is defined broadly to include loss of role, loss of physical health, loss of ability, loss of relationships, and ultimately loss of one's own life.

Role change is a central issue facing many elderly persons. As one ages, losses in social roles and status can occur. These may be the result of retirement, a change in income, decline in health, death of a spouse or other family member. Although roles are added and lost throughout life, there is a net decline in the total number of roles played out after the middle years (29). Role loss is more consequential in the elderly because often there are no readily available replacements for the loss. Furthermore, there is often an accompanying decrease in responsibilities, status, and activity.

Another potential loss facing old people is loss of the producer role through retirement. "One out of five older men work in contrast to the turn of the century when two out of three men who were 65 years of age or older were still working" (30). Accompanying retirement there may be an associated decrease in social status, income, self-esteem and activity level. The decrease or loss of income from retirement frequently negatively impacts the elderly. Retirement income drops to one-half of pre-retirement income and many elderly in this century live below poverty guidelines (30).

For many men, work is the central role in their lives and loss of this role can be crucial. It has been shown that the effects of a forced age-related retirement are more deleterious than the effects of a chosen, planned retirement. However, women seem to cope better with retirement because they have often maintained a dual role of career person and homemaker and continue the homemaker role into retirement, thus eliminating the major impact of loss of the work role.

Another change may occur in the areas of intimacy and sexuality. Contrary to popular belief the need for intimacy and sexual expression continues throughout the life cycle. The age-related sexual patterns of men and women are different. Men reach the peak of their sexual activity in young adulthood and then experience a slow steady decline with increasing age. However, sexuality in women follows a different pattern. Women do not experience the same decline as men and even though they experience menopause in middle age, it does not mean that they cease sexual activity. Many couples enjoy sexual expression well into old age. Attitudes toward sexuality in the aged often reflect past patterns, health status, and attitudes toward aging in general.

The greatest loss experienced by humans is the death of a loved one. The loss of a spouse is stressful and is associated with increased incidence of illness and death in the bereaved. Death of a spouse or a friend severs many ties to the world around an elderly person leading to further alienation from an active society. This is probably more true for men who are more dependent on the social skills of the wife. Death of a spouse may occur at all ages; however, its occurrence is most frequent among aged females. The acute symptoms of bereavement last one to three months, but the effects of the death continue to be felt for a much longer period of time.

It seems that older adults are better prepared for their own deaths and have less fear about it than younger groups (31). Often, the elderly show more concern about the death of a loved one than they do their own death. Views of a death seem to reflect one's views throughout the adaptive processes of one's life.

Adaptation is a dynamic process requiring adjustment to the biological and psychological changes related to aging, as well as accomodating to the demands of a changing society. Successful adaptation requires a redefinition of social role, a substitution of new interests and activities, a reassessment of the criteria for self-evaluation and a reintegration of values and life goals (32).

REFERENCES

1. Shock, NW: In *Proceedings of Seminars*, Jeffers, FC (Ed.), Center for the Study of Aging and Human Development, Duke University, Durham, NC, 1962, pp. 123-140.

2. Shock, NW: Aging of Regulatory Mechanisms. In *Fundamentals of Geriatric Medicine*, Cape, RDT; Coe, RM; Rossman, I (Eds.). New York: Raven Press, 1983.

3. Goldman, R: Decline in Organ Function with Aging. In *Clinical Geriatrics*, 2nd Edition, Rossman, I (Ed.). Philadelphia: JB Lippincott Co., 1979.

4. Miall, WE; Ashcroft, MT; Lovell, HG, *et. al.*: A Longitudinal Study of the Decline of Adult Height with Age in Two Welsh Communities. *Hum Biol, 39:*445, 1967.

5. Rossman, I: The Anatomy of Aging. In *Clinical Geriatrics*, 2nd Edition, Rossman, I (Ed.). Philadelphia: JB Lippincott, Co., 1979.

6. De Vries, HA: Tips on Prescribing Exercise Regimens for Your Older Patients. *Geriatrics, 34:*75, 1979.

7. Finch, CS; Hayflick, L: *Handbook of the Biology of Aging*. New York: Van Nostrand Reinhold Co., 1977.

8. Yu, BP; Masoro, EJ; Murata, I, *et al.*: Life span study of SPF Fischer 344 male rats fed ad libitum or restricted diets: longevity, lean body mass and disease. *J Gerontol, 37:*130, 1982.

9. Masoro, EJ; Compton, C; Yu, BP, *et al.*: Temporal and Compositional Dietary Restrictions Modulate Age-related Changes in Serum Lipids. *J Nutr, 113:*880, 1983.

10. Weindruck, R; Wolford, RL: Dietary restriction in mice beginning at 1 year of age: effect on life span and spontaneous cancer incidence. *Science, 215:*1415, 1982.

11. Hazzard, WR: Dyslipoproteinemia and Obesity. In *Geriatric Medicine: Medical, Psychiatric and Pharmacological Topics*, Vol I, Cassel, C and Walsh, J (Eds.). New York: Springer-Verlag, 1984, pp. 472-484.

12. Andres, R: Aging, Diabetes and Obesity: Standards of Normality. *Mt Sinai J Med, 48:*489, 1981.

13. Honch, GW; Spitzer, RM: Radiographic Aids to the Diagnosis of Dementia in the Elderly. *Sem Neurol, 1:*53, 1981.

14. Brody, H; Vijayashankar, N: Anatomic Changes in the Nervous System. In *Handbook of the Biology of Aging*, Finch, E and Hayflick, L (Eds.). New York: Van Nostrand Reinhold, 1977, pp. 241-262.

15. Schneck, SA: Aging of the Nervous System and Dementia. In *Clinical Internal Medicine in the Aged*, Schrier, RW (Ed.). Philadelphia: WB Saunders Co., 1982, pp. 41–42.

16. Rowe, JW; Besdine, RW: *Health and Disease in Old Age.* Boston: Little, Brown and Co, 1982, p. 165.

17. Rowe, JW; Andres, R; Tobin, JD, *et al.*: The effect of age on creatinine clearance in man: A cross-sectional and longitudinal study. *J Gerontol*, *31:*155, 1976.

18. Epstein, M; Hollenberg, NK: Age as a Determinant of Renal Sodium Conservation in Normal Men. *J Lab Clin Med*, *97:*411, 1976.

19. Gerber, JG: Drug Usage in the Elderly. In *Clinical Internal Medicine in the Aged*, Schrier, R (Ed.). Philadelphia: WB Saunders Co, 1982.

20. Botwinick, J: Intellectual Abilities. In *Handbook of the Psychology of Aging*, Birren, JE and Schoie KW (Eds.). New York: Van Nostrand Reinhold, 1977.

21. Hodkinson, HM: *An Outline of Geriatrics.* New York: Grune and Stratton, 1981.

22. Atchley, RC: *The Social Forces in Later Life*, 3ed Edition. Belmont, CA: Wadsworth, Publishing Company, 1980.

23. Storandt, M: Psychological Aspects. In *Care of the Geriatric Patient*, 6th Edition, Steinberg, FV (Ed.). St. Louis: The CV Mosby Company, 1983, pp. 417–428.

24. Storandt, M: Age, ability level and method of administering and scoring the WAIS. *J of Gerontol*, *32:*175–179, 1977.

25. Wells, Thelma: *Aging and Health Promotion.* Rockville, MD: Aspin Systems Corporation, 1982.

26. Howieson, D: Cognitive Changes in the Elderly. Lecture presented at Veterans Administration Medical Center, Portland, OR, 2/9/84.

27. Cumming, E; Henry, WR: *Growing Old: The Process of Disengagement.* New York: Basic Books, 1961.

28. Butler, R; Lewis, M: *Aging and Mental Health.* St. Louis, CV Mosby Co.

29. Buhler, C: The general structure of the human life cycle, In *The Course of Human Life: A Study of Goals in the Human Perspective*, Buhler, C and Massarik, F (Eds.). New York: Springer-Verlag, 1968.

30. Blumenthal, M: Psychiatric Aspects. In *Care of the Geriatric Patient*, 6th Edition, Steinberg, FV (Ed.). St. Louis: CV Mosby Co, 1983, pp. 429–449.

31. Bengston, V: *The Social Psychology of Aging.* Indianapolis: Bobbs-Merrill, 1973.

32. Clark, M; Anderson, B: *Culture and Aging.* Springfield, IL: Chas C Thomas, 1967.

CHAPTER 3

HEALTH PROMOTION AND PREVENTIVE STRATEGIES

Many preventive strategies used to enhance health should be started early in life. However, preventive medicine is equally important in the elderly, a discussion of health promotion and prevention in the frail elderly may appear incongruent, yet it is probably more critical at this stage of life to prevent disability, social isolation, falls, fractures, urinary incontinence, confusion, depression and deterioration of an existing disorder. Preventive medicine in the conventional sense is usually focused on prevention of disease before it occurs through immunizations, dietary prevention for atherosclerosis, lifestyle changes to reduce obesity, and to prevent lung or cardiovascular problems by eliminating cigarette smoking or liver disease by interdicting drinking of alcoholic beverages. Furthermore, prevention in the elderly is intended to slow or forestall decline of functional activity through an anticipatory approach to block progression of diseases, and consequences of medication use or other iatrogenic problems (1, 2). The practice of prospective or anticipatory medicine to prevent irreversible and often fatal consequences in the frail elderly illustrates the principle that prevention transcends treatment of complications. To anticipate complications and prevent them is a practical everyday management strategy that fosters independence. Many aspects of prevention have been discussed in other chapters such as prevention of falls, incontinence, adverse drug reactions, constipation, osteoporosis, hypo and hyperthermia to name a few.

WELLNESS

The wellness movement promotes lifestyle activities that enhance health; a focus on well-being rather than disease. It is a

41

concept based on self-responsibility for our own health and implies that people become well-informed about healthy practices (3). Behavioral strategies to achieve wellness consist of prospective planning to reduce risk factors that most likely will lead to disability and even death (4). Paradoxically, some of these risk factors are the unhealthy habits marketed in our society with which most people identify and, therefore, continue to smoke, drink, eat too much and exercise too little. If people are to be responsible for their own health they must be taught how to be responsible and health care providers must provide factual data to overcome the constant bombardment of advertising that reinforce bad habits (5). Behavioral strategies to improve our health should begin early in life. Cessation of smoking, using alcoholic beverages in moderation, use of seat belts, appropriate exercise, low salt, sugar, cholesterol and saturated fat diets, and adopting a relaxed convivial lifestyle, in the aggregate decrease the risk of heart disease, stroke, lung cancer, chronic obstructive lung disease, liver cirrhosis and accidental injuries. Emphasis on wellness is an attractive and seemingly obvious concept for healthy living, but the danger is that some people are caught up with the extremes which border on quackery. Trendy modalities should not be unquestionably over-indulged in without more factual data. In the extreme, elderly people must be protected from enthusiasts who endorse an irresponsible acceptance of self-accountability for health even for cancer or overwhelming infection to the exclusion of physician intervention; e.g., an antiphysician posture. However, faith is an important ingredient in healing and reasonable self-responsible attitudes toward even serious disease may enable us to better accept our discomfort. Health providers should not expect uninformed consumers to accept responsibility beyond their limits. But it is logical that informed individuals accept some responsibility for maintenance of their health whether it be lifestyle or compliance with appropriate medications.

NUTRITION

Contrary to general belief, nutrition is not a major problem in most healthy elderly persons. One can expect, however, nutritional problems in the frail elderly who by virtue of their long existence have accumulated more disability. There is a broad range of conditions in this age group that affect nutritional status. Some of these factors are apathy, loneliness, depression, dementia, limited mobility from physical disability, poor vision, infections, chronic illness, swallowing problems, drugs, alcoholism, poor dietary habits, dietary fads, poverty, lack of transportation, among others. Immobility fosters dependency and increases the risk of poor nutrition. Undernutrition occurs in 10% of old people with a variety of disabling conditions that render them housebound (6). The loss of spouse and friends dampens motivation to prepare a full meal, especially for those who have been unaccustomed to preparing their own meals. Nonetheless, we must avoid sweeping generalities since some socially isolated older people cook satisfactory meals even on a hot plate.

Energy requirements vary according to health and mobility. As we grow older our total energy needs are less because physical activity decreases. Reduction of high caloric foods but also recognizing the need for protein, vitamins and minerals in the diet will prevent malnutrition. Caloric intake should be adjusted to a level that prevents both excessive overweight and underweight, both of which are associated with disease. Loss of weight secondary to anorexia (Table 3.1) is a common problem in the frail elderly. Ensuring that sufficient nutrients are consumed by the patient is often a monumental task requiring the expertise of the interdisciplinary team.

There are many factors affecting adequate nutrition. Absence of teeth or loose fitting dentures prevents proper chewing of many

TABLE 3.1
FACTORS CAUSING LOSS OF APPETITE

Drugs	Diseases
Digitalis	Malignancy
Aspirin	Chronic renal insufficiency
Nonsteroidal anti-inflammatory	Congestive heart failure
Reserpine	Infection
Amphetamines	Hyperthyroidism
Theophylline	Gall bladder disease
Depression	Addison's disease
Living alone	Disease producing dysphagia
Fecal impaction	

solid foods such as raw fruits, vegetables, and meat. A stroke or other neurological disorders may cause swallowing difficulties, including choking which occurs predominantly with liquids. In aged persons, a diminished sense of taste and smell frequently dampens the stimulus to eat. Other older people often have diminished saliva and gastric digestive juices that may be further aggravated by anticholinergic drugs which dries the mouth and diminishes taste. Adequate fluid intake is an important aspect of nutrition since dehydration from inadequate fluid intake can cause confusion, weakness, and poor dietary intake. Many drugs diminish appetite (Table 3.1) and lead to poor nutrition.

The elderly often have problems with food preparation and resources to purchase food are inadequate. Older people with a poor income may have inadequate cooking facilities, thereby limiting the type and variety of food that can be prepared. Immobility and lack of exercise can diminish appetite. Physical impairments from a stroke or arthritis or other conditions may interfere with the preparation of meals or be an obstacle in getting to the store to purchase foods. A nourishing meal may be replaced by tea and toast or coffee and doughnuts when a person living alone has little incentive to prepare an adequate meal.

One of the dangers of nutrition fadism is a tendency for people to obtain information from radical health food advocates regarding decisions concerning diet. Unfortunately, considerable misinformation dressed up with eye–catching slogans is contradictory to traditional information given by nutritional experts. There is much unknown in the nutritional field and it is because of these gaps in our knowledge that health food enthusiasts seize the opportunity to widely promote their claims to those most susceptible to exploitation. People have been persuaded that life can be prolonged, arthritis cured and dementia prevented with special diets, mineral and vitamin supplements. Persuasive tactics assure us that megavitamins and natural rather than synthetic foods, are dietary panaceas. These assurances decieve the disabled elderly who are looking for ways to slow their failing health or to prolong life. But to date, there is no evidence that any diet will perform the miracles attributed to them or that they will prolong life.

Vitamins. Prodigious advertising and the vast consumption of vitamins by the young and the old gives a false impression that vitamin deficiency is widespread in the United States. However, certain subgroups of our population are more likely to develop hypovitaminosis. The frail elderly are particularly at risk of developing vitamin deficiency because of severely restricted diets. Nonetheless, many elderly people who use vitamin supplements have adequate dietary intake. There are some observers who state that oral supplementation is inadequate for the elderly person and suggest that intramuscular vitamin therapy is necessary for preventing or correcting hypovitaminosis (7). Obviously, further research is needed to support this approach before it can be recommended. The elderly population is particularly vulnerable to misconceptions regarding vitamin supplements. Non-specific symptons such as fatigue, weakness, and lack of energy may be the result of vitamin deficiency, however, they are also symptoms of problems which commonly occur in many older people who do not have vitamin deficiency. Since the elderly are usually on fixed or reduced incomes, the cost of vitamin supplements is an important issue. A recent survey of older people showed that almost 50% used a vitamin or mineral supplement, most taking a multivitamin (8). The use of supplements increases progressively with age so that 60% over the age of 80 years use vitamins (8). As physical disabilities become more numerous or symptomatic, the elderly person is progressively more receptive to information about products promising relief of symptoms. Older people use supplements because they preceive added health benefits from these products. Two common misbeliefs about consuming vitamins are that the higher the cost the better the quality, and the greater the amount taken the greater the physiologic benefits. Counseling elderly patients about nutritious food and dietary supplements, therefore, should receive high priority in health care.

Vitamins are divided into nine water-soluble (B_1, B_2, B_6, B_{12}, C, niacin, folate, biotin, and pantothenic acid) and four fat-soluble agents (A, D, E and K). The recommended daily allowance (RDA) is set at levels two to six times higher than the MDR (minimal daily requirement) which represents an adequate intake to prevent deficiency. The RDA for water-soluble vitamins range from 0.5 mg to 100 mg a day. Generally speaking, most vitamins especially water-soluble vitamins are nontoxic even in large doses since the body is believed to excrete excesses in the urine. There have been adverse responses, however, to large doses of vitamin C, niacin, vitamin B_6 (Pyridoxine) and folic acid. The fat-soluble vitamins A and D are definitely toxic in large amounts. Vitamin A toxicity classically presents with increased intracranial pressure although the reason for the increased intracranial pressure is unclear (9). Fortunately, symptoms and signs resolve spontaneously after cessation of the vitamin A intake. Disturbances of skin and hair, sleep disturbances, loss of appetite, weight loss, hepatosplenomegaly, elevated serum alkaline phosphatase and occasional hypercalcemia may develop (9).

Vitamin D toxicity occurs with doses as low as 10,000 I.U. daily over a period of several months. More commonly, daily ingestion of 50,000–500,000 I.U. for several years precedes toxicity. Hypercalcemia accounts for symptoms of anorexia, weight loss, nausea, vomiting, constipation, apathy, weakness, fatigue, mental confusion, polyuria, polydipsia, hyperphosphatemia, metastatic calcifications in soft tissues and bone pain (9). Even after discontinuation of vitamin D adverse symptoms persist for as long as 22 months.

Megavitamins. "If a little is good, more is better" is a common misbelief not only in the taking of any medication, but in the consuming of vitamins. Megadose or megavitamin therapy is a regimen that involves the ingestion of supraphysiologic amounts of vitamins. In general, ten or more times the recommended dietary allowance (RDA) represents megavitamin therapy. The benefits of megavitamin therapy have been exaggerated by enthusiasts as a nostrum to prevent disorders in the healthy and to cure disabilities of the infirm. This form of therapy has been endorsed to prevent or cure colds, infections, arthritis, cancer, and even to postpone aging, but without much supportive data to substantiate these claims (9). Vitamin and mineral therapy is a two billion dollar a year industry and health professionals should be concerned about the cost and even possible danger associated with indiscriminate use of vitamin supplements in the elderly. An example of a serious toxic effect of a vitamin is the progressive ataxia with severe impairment of position and vibratory sense after consumption of $\geq$ 2 gram doses of pyridoxine daily recently reported in seven young adult patients (10). Recovery gradually occurred after stopping the pyridoxine. In an elderly population these symptoms could easily be ascribed to old age, or to a neurological disease. Animal studies using high doses of pyridoxine have shown a progressively unsteady gait due to a sensory neuronopathy.

Vitamin C is used frequently in megadoses. Vitamin C enthusiasts recommend it for a wide variety of conditions. Claims of a reduced incidence and severity of viral, bacterial, or fungal infection, prevention of venous thrombosis, atherosclerosis, and complications of diabetes mellitus, promotion of wound healing, and enhancement of mental alertness have been promoted but not scientifically validated (9). Diarrhea with abdominal cramps may occur with the ingestion of more than 1 gram of vitamin C per day. Patients known to develop kidney stones should not take megadoses of vitamin C since there is a theoretical possibility that increased urinary oxalate excretion and uricosuria may lead to nephrolithiasis. This is not firmly established, however. The strong reducing properties of vitamin C may cause false positive results with urine glucose tests in diabetics.

Folate Deficiency

Both folate and vitamin B_{12} deficiencies cause a similar type of megaloblastic anemia with peripheral blood morphology that is indistinguishable. Nutritional folate deficiency is more common than vitamin B_{12} deficiency in the elderly as a consequence of poor dietary intake. The dietary intake of folate in the elderly is usually less than 200 μg per day and 30% of elderly have an intake less than 100 μg per day. The recommended dietary allowance for folate is 400 μg per day for the elderly which is much greater than actually needed since even 150 μg grams per day may be protective against folate deficiency (11). Folates are found in nearly all raw foods such as green vegetables, liver, kidneys, and dairy products; but excessive cooking readily destroys folates. Elderly people whose daily diet does not include fresh or fresh frozen uncooked fruit, fruit juice or fresh lightly cooked vegetables are at risk to develop folate deficiency.

Using the serum folate level of $\langle$ 3 ng/ml as an indication for deficiency several studies have observed up to 10% of urban and rural low income elderly have a high risk for folate deficiency (11). Institutionalized and hospitalized elderly in the United States are at high risk for developing folate deficiency. Almost 20% of all nursing home residents and up to 34% of residents over 75 years of age have low serum folate levels. Folate deficiency is, therefore, more of a problem in the low income elderly and hospitalized and institutionalized patients. There is an increased prevalence of folate deficiency in alcoholics who have been eating poorly. It occurs more frequently with wine and whiskey drinkers rather than with beer drinkers since the former contains practically no folate while there is ample folate in beer. The addition of folic acid to alcoholic beverages has even been recommended to prevent deficiency in alcoholics. There is a high incidence of alcoholism among the elderly, much of which is not recognized as a problem.

A low serum folate is a common finding in elderly patients admitted to hospitals or institutions. This is largely due to alcoholism associated with poor eating habits, as well as diseases and drugs which interfere with the intake and utilization of folate. Elderly people who develop loss of appetite due to illness, drugs, or depression may have a serum folate ⟨ 3 ng/ml early in hospitalization. An individual with anorexia may develop a low serum folate in approximately two weeks. The serum folate quickly returns to normal with an adequate diet. In this situation the red cell folate determination is a better index of tissue folate stores. An erythrocyte folate level of less than 140 ng/ml is indicative of folate deficiency.

Neurological and psychiatric symptoms occur with vitamin B_{12} deficiency, although the severity does not correlate with the degree of anemia (12). Peripheral neuropathy and lateral and posterior spinal cord lesions are complications of vitamin B_{12} deficiency that should be prevented. Furthermore, personality changes, confusion, dementia, and depression may partially or completely resolve with vitamin B_{12} therapy if due to a deficiency. However, vitamin B_{12} deficiency may coexist with senile dementia of Alzheimer's type (SDAT) or multi-infarction dementia. Therapy with vitamin B_{12} may improve physical and mental activity by reversing the metabolic abnormality and correcting the anemia, but cannot be expected to improve the basic underlying SDAT or multi-infarct dementia (13).

On the other hand, folate deficiency usually does not produce peripheral neuropathy itself but it may occur in some patients in whom the folate deficiency is due to alcoholism. Folate deficiency occurs in patients with dementia or depression, but is related to the anorexia and bizarre eating habits associated with these disorders. Folate deficiency, however, may be implicated in the etiology of depression by interference with the synthesis of dopamine and serotonin, which stems from the folate deficiency (12, 14). Yet, there is little substantial evidence that folate deficiency itself is a cause of dementia, although any anemia may worsen an existing dementia. Therefore, the correction of the anemia related to folate deficiency may improve some features of the underlying dementia.

Iron Deficiency

Iron deficiency anemia is the most common nutritional anemia in the elderly. Mean iron intake is adequate until the age of 75 but little is known beyond this age (15). The recommended daily allowance (RDA) for iron is 10 mg of which approximately 1 mg is absorbed. Although older people have poorer diets, the intake of iron is achieved by increasing the iron nutrient density from the usual normal of about 6 mg of elemental iron per 1000 kcal to nearly 8 mg of iron per 1000 kcal (15). In the frail elderly with a greatly reduced caloric intake, the average iron intake may fall below the RDA, but iron stores are lost at a slow rate. Some groups of elderly may be at high risk for iron deficiency, such as nursing home patients, those living alone, especially those with physical disabilities, and those who take few hot meals. Nonetheless, the average total iron intake is adequate for most elderly Americans. Iron from animal tissue is better absorbed than iron from vegetables. Vegetable sources may be high in iron content, but the iron is poorly absorbed because of inhibitors to iron absorption such as phosphates and phytates which occur in plants. Although spinach may contain ample iron, it is not as good a dietary source of iron as traditionally believed. Tea is an inhibitor of iron absorption and some elderly people drink large quantities of tea daily which produces iron deficiency, especially if the diet consists mainly of vegetables (16).

The popular explanation that iron deficiency anemia in an elderly person is related to a poor diet is unacceptable unless an evaluation for a bleeding lesion has been completed. A concomitant bleeding lesion is often the cause of iron deficiency even in patients who have a poor dietary history (17). It is, therefore, axiomatic that in an elderly person with an iron deficiency anemia a search for an underlying lesion is mandatory. On the other hand a dietary deficiency may be a contributing factor. Iron losses in older men and women are no greater than in younger men, therefore, requirements for older people are no greater than adult men, but are lower than for children and menstruating women.

Zinc

Zinc deficiency in the elderly is due to combined effects of diet, disease, alcohol and medications. Elderly people who cannot afford meat, poultry, fish, milk, cheese, and eggs are at risk to develop zinc deficiency. Foods that reduce zinc absorption are cereals containing phytate such as oatmeal and high fiber bran cereals. Diseases leading to zinc deficiency are hepatic and renal disease and disorders associated with muscle wasting. Alcoholics are prone to develop zinc deficiency. Drugs which increase renal loss of zinc such as diuretics and digitalis glycosides may be implicated with zinc deficiency.

Loss of taste may be due to zinc deficiency, however, this is a common finding in older people most often unrelated to zinc. Some studies support the role of zinc in wound healing. Zinc is considered important in immune functions of the elderly, but our knowledge is still limited.

Protein–Calorie Malnutrition (PCM)

Insufficient protein intake, increased requirements, or excessive protein loss can lead to protein–calorie malnutrition. It occurs more frequently in hospitalized and nursing home patients (19–22), usually secondary to an underlying disease. It often results from low food intake secondary to anorexia (Table 3.1). Economic factors, severe depression, decreased ability to cook meals, loneliness, and isolation severely compromise the diet of indigent elderly while immobility is responsible for muscle and bone loss, factors that encourage development of PCM. Both PCM and the aging process itself cause similar reductions in muscle mass and hematopoetic function (22). The disorder is frequently overlooked, especially in hospitals and nursing homes and may be misdiagnosed as failure to thrive or cachexia of heart, lung, or liver disease.

In the management of elderly patients, particularly the frail elderly, PCM may be responsible for inadequate responses to stress, delayed wound healing and increasing incidence of infections (22). An impairment in cell–mediated immunity occurs, with alteration of T cells. There is a reduction of neutrophil response to infection. A decreased ability of early bone marrow stem cells to proliferate contributes significantly to anemia, an early manifestation of PCM. Aging itself causes similar changes in immunity and suppression of bone marrow cell proliferation but to lesser extent than PCM. The additive effect of PCM superimposed on the decline from aging increases morbidity and mortality.

Often attributed to other causes, confusion or altered mental status is a frequent symptom of PCM. Dehydration is the most common cause of an acute confusional state in the elderly and patients with PCM often have an inadequate fluid intake so that dehydration may be the mechanism for the confusion. There is a significant weight loss from protein malnutrition. Depression is often suspected. Infections are often present such as pneumonia or urinary tract infections.

Signs of cachexia are emaciation, loss of subcutaneous fat, loss of lean body mass, brittle hair, ridged nails and sometimes skin rash of lower legs. It is often stated that a low serum albumin is common with advanced age. It appears, however, that the low serum albumin is related to malnutrition (22–24) or underlying disease rather than being age related. The history of recent weight loss with a serum albumin of less than 3.5 mg/dl (not due to hepatic failure or renal disease), associated often with anemia, lymphocytopenia, and anergy to skin tests with candida and mumps antigens, support the diagnosis (22). Serum transferrin levels less than 170 μg/dl is similarly indicative of protein depletion although it is influenced by infection and body iron status.

Treatment of PCM consists of management of infection, control of blood pressure, and correction of fluid and electrolyte problems. Only a small percentage of elderly subjects with PCM can correct the nutritional deficiency by oral intake which consists of calorie and nutrient dense foods. Many need an enteral form of hyperalimentation. With this therapy, weight is gained, serum albumin increases, anemia is corrected, lymphocyte counts return to normal, total iron binding capacity increases, anergy disappears, and there is an increase in bone marrow activity (22). Prolonged nutritional support with hyperalimentation by means of nasogastric tube and intensive rehabilitation results in remarkable improvement in nutritional status.

The use of small, soft nasogastric and nasojejunal tubes for enteral hyperalimentation provides a safe and relatively comfortable way to feed patients. Sometimes remarkable changes in behavior, physical ability, strength and mental outlook occur in patients who are rapidly declining, depressed, wish to die, confused, or refuse physical therapy, within 7 to 10 days of nutritional support (19). There are no clear criteria to select which patients will respond to nutritional intervention and until guidelines are available health care providers must use available evidence to make decisions about which patients will benefit and conversely which patients will unnecessarily have their lives prolonged.

Role of the Dietician
on the Geriatric Interdisciplinary Team

The dietician has a responsibility to assess the patient to identify those at particular risk of nutritional inadequacy, to determine nutritional plans, supervise food intake of institutionalized patients, teach members of the interdisciplinary team, educate the patient and family/caregivers and work with other members of the interdisciplinary team to improve the patient's nutritional status not only in the hospital but to make dietary recommendations for whatever level of placement ensues.

The role of the dietician is to:

1. Assess nutritional needs of older patients.
2. Identify patients at nutritional risk: A) Use calorie counts, B) laboratory data, and C) anthropometric measurements.
3. Consult with other members of the interdisciplinary team and make recommendations for dietary or feeding changes to improve nutrition status.
4. Determine and recommend special dietary needs.
5. Coordinate with other team members on specific feeding problems such as, speech and occupational therapists, and nursing personnel about swallowing problems.
6. Instructing patients and families/caregivers on any special diet at time of hospital discharge.
7. Develop educational materials specific to geriatric nutrition education.
8. Coordinate any special nutritional needs for nursing home placement with Social Work Service prior to patient discharge.
9. Discuss dietery problems at ward rounds and interdisciplinary team meetings.
10. Participate in Geriatric seminars.
11. Serve as role model to dietetic intern.
12. Provide outpatient nutrition follow-up in the Geriatric Clinic.

EXERCISE

After age 30, muscle atrophy, bone loss and instability causes a decline in function. However, disuse from a sedentary lifestyle is also a major contributing factor. Obviously, the antidote is exercise, especially of the aerobic type. Aerobic exercise is a rhythmic constant, not overly strenuous movement of large muscles over an extended period of time in which the oxygen demand of the muscle does not exceed the supply. This activity promotes an increased heart rate, cardiac output and oxygen consumption with a goal to improve cardiovascular fitness. Examples of aerobic exercises are running, cycling, swimming, racket sports, handball, aerobic dance and cross country skiing. In contrast, anaerobic exercise consists of brief high exertion or strenuous activity which results in an oxygen debt as the oxygen lags behind the demand. This usually involves isometric exercises for muscle strengthening and include such activities as push-ups, weight lifting, leg lifts and hand grip exercise.

During physical activity, blood flow through muscles may increase 15 to 20 times over resting values, coronary artery blood flow increases but blood flow through abdominal organs is greatly reduced. The heart rate rises, pulmonary ventilation increases and systolic blood pressure climbs (25-27). As effort intensifies more oxygen is consumed along with the increasing heart rate. But both maximal heart rate (the fastest your heart can beat) and maximal oxygen consumption decline with advancing age (27, 28). This means that the older you are the slower your heart beats during maximum exercise and less oxygen is available to muscles. A decrease in maximum heart rate does not hinder mild exercise but with stressful physical activity the heart is unable to deliver enough blood to supply sufficient oxygen to muscles. When exercise is prescribed, it should be performed at the appropriate heart rate. A rough approximation of maximal heart rate which can be used as a general guide is calculated by a formula (220 − age). Exercise is initially prescribed to keep the heart rate 20-30% above the resting heart rate and with conditioning exercise is increased in small increments but keeping the heart rate below 70% of the maximum heart rate.

In addition, respiratory changes which occur with advancing age decreases the oxygen supply. Vital capacity, the amount of air a person can exhale after a deep breath is reduced. Stiffening of the chest wall in an elderly person results in considerably greater muscular effort to move air in and out of the lungs and less air is moved. An elderly person, therefore, has some limitation in the ability to carry oxygen from the ambient air to muscle cells due to aging changes in both the heart and respiratory system. Heart or lung disease further reduces the ability to supply oxygen during increased physical activity.

Loss of muscle fibers (3–5% per decade after age 30) with inactivity during advancing age leads to loss of muscle tone, strength and endurance. Muscles can be strengthened, range of joint motion and flexibility improved with regular exercise. Older people who exercise regularly develop increased muscle mass, stronger and larger bones (physical activity diminishes rate of decline of bone which is especially important for postmenopausal women), show improvement in pulse rate, blood pressure, flexibility, coordination and balance, endurance, physical work capacity and in feelings of well–being. Physical training reduces weight particularly by decreasing the body fat, and reduces systolic pressure (25, 26). Sustained aerobic exercise lowers cholesterol levels and there is some evidence that it may also raise the level of protective high density lipoprotein levels (25, 26). Regular aerobic exercise produces slow weight loss but as body fat declines, muscle mass increases and because muscle is denser than fat the net weight loss may be slight. Remember, too, that is takes 35 miles of walking or jogging to use up the calories present in one pound of adipose tissue (25). Therefore, exercise alone without attention to dietary intake will not cause significant weight reduction.

Exercise has other possible beneficial results. Regular exercise is reported to have a tranquilizing effect on the individual (29). It has also been thought to ameliorate mild depression. After exercise most people will claim that they feel much better and elevated beta endorphin levels have been suggested as a possible explanation. Endorphins are hormones produced by the body which inhibit pain. Exercise also increases stress on the bone and conversely, inactivity has been correlated with bone loss; exercise has been used to prevent osteoporosis although other factors are important.

Before undertaking exercises, the frail elderly should be taught not only about the benefits but also the risks of habitual exercise. It is particularly the sedentary disabled frail elderly who must avoid overexertion in an exercise program (Figure 3.1). Patients with severe heart disease and congestive heart failure, heart muscle irritability, unstable angina, aortic aneurysm, uncontrolled diabetes, severe obstructive pulmonary disease or uncontrolled seizure disorders should be cautioned about exercise. For many frail elderly people walking is a splendid form of exercise. Brisk walking at five miles an hour or walking one mile in 12

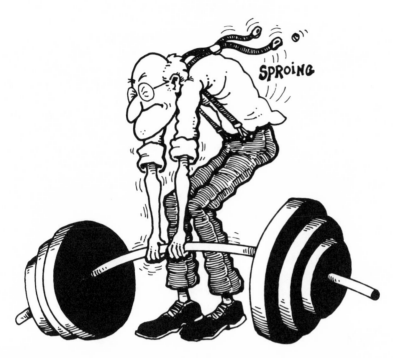

Figure 3.1. Pumping iron or pumping trouble — over-reaching our limitations. The athletes' motto "no pain, no gain" is unrealistic for the elderly.

minutes will maintain fitness. Some exercises such as swimming, walking, dancing are well suited to the physical limitations of the elderly. At least three sessions per week for at least 30 minutes of activity is a goal that should be attained. Some may never attain it. However, an untrained individual must progress slowly and each exercise session should be proceeded by a five to ten minute warm-up and followed by a similar cool-down period. Stretching exercises, gentle calisthenics and walking are prescribed for these purposes. Walking is excellent for leg strength and endurance. Chair exercises can be performed by most older adults (27). These can be programmed as rhythmic exercises for both the lower and upper extremities. Less vigorous recreational activities can often be tailored for the elderly. For frail older people or those who are bedridden short periods of stretching or flexing exercises may be the upper limit of tolerance.

IMMUNIZATIONS

Two serious causes of respiratory infections are pneumococcal pneumonia and influenza (flu). Both diseases are preventable by immunizaiton. These are the two most common immunizations in the elderly and should not be confused. Pneumonia is the fifth leading cause of death in the elderly. Pneumococcal pneumonia is a common and serious disease in older people. There is an increasing prevalence of pneumonia with advancing age. Mortality is five to ten times higher in the elderly.

A pneumococcal vaccine is now available with 23 of the commonest pneumococcal serotypes. The vaccine is administered as a single 0.5 ml injection and should be given to all people over 65 years of age. Existing data indicates that no individual will benefit from revaccination and that substantial risk of adverse reactions occur with revaccination (29).

Most patients who die of influenza infection are elderly. The mortality rate from influenza in the elderly is twenty times that seen in younger patients. Influenza occurs as both endemic and epidemic disease in the community but has also been shown to be associated with outbreaks in long-term care facilities. Vaccination results in less severe illness and lower mortality. Immunization is recommended for virtually all patients over 65 (30). Annual influenza immunizations are strongly recommended for all older people.

Tetanus is a disease that occurs more frequently in the elderly and serious consideration should be given to immunizations (30). Comprehensive programs of tetanus–diphtheria toxoid are given to children but only a small portion of individuals over 60 years of age have serum antitoxin levels which are protective against tetanus. Older individuals have a diminished antibody level against diphtheria toxin. A large number of men have been vaccinated against tetanus during military service in World War II. However, many elderly, particularly elderly women are unprotected and tetanus is a serious disease which often ends with death of the patients. If elderly persons have not been immunized against tetanus they should receive primary tetanus–diphtheria toxoid and should receive boosters every ten years.

ALCOHOLISM

As people age, the number of abstainers increases and the total amount of alcohol consumed decreases. Men continue to drink at the same rate through the sixth decade but there is a drop in the prevalence of heavy drinking after 75 years of age (31). Nonetheless, alcoholism is more prevalent in the elderly than formerly realized. It is estimated that there are approximately three million older people over age 60 who are alcoholics (32). It is difficult to obtain accurate figures because there is a high rate of denial of drinking alcohol in the older segment of the population. Of those who seek medical attention, 10–15% have an alcohol–related problem (33). There are two types of alcoholics in the elderly population. Most alcoholics have been drinking most of their lives and continue to drink when they become older. There is an increased incidence of accidents, brain and liver damage in this population. Many heavy drinkers do not live to an old age but significant numbers capable of enduring these hardships survive to old age. On the other hand, about one–third of alcoholics are late–onset who begin drinking as a solution to loneliness, depression, marital problems, bereavement, and economic hardship (24). There is an increasing number of women surfacing as late–onset alcoholics. Alcohol use is sometimes concealed in older people because they are outside the mainstream of social activity, live alone, do not work, and rarely have automobile accidents because they drive only short distances and do not frequent bars and lounges, and, therefore, are not often taken into custody by the police.

Age seemingly decreases tolerance to alcohol and frail old people are especially susceptible to alcohol. Alcohol is cleared more slowly from the body in older people. Therefore, smaller amounts may produce severe consequences in physically or mentally debilitated elderly people. Alcohol is often a reason for falling, producing fractures and other head and leg injuries. Older people may not tell their doctor about consuming alcohol which, in fact, may be responsible for their episodes of falling. A patient with mild or moderate dementia may become confused when drinking even small amounts of alcohol. There is also a risk that an older alcoholic may be mistakenly diagnosed as having dementia (35). The health care provider should always be alert to alcoholism as a reason to account for falls and for confusional episodes. Alcoholism may cause confusion, disorientation, and paranoia which, in turn, causes difficulties in family relationships or may be responsible for alienating friends and associates. Often depression or hostility accompanies alcoholism. Older alcoholics may seclude themselves over a prolonged period, make mistakes in shopping or handling of money, and develop erratic eating and sleeping habits. Alcohol can contribute to poor dietary habits and lead to malnutrition. Folate deficiency anemia is related to alcoholism. Older people in nursing homes drink to make institutional life bearable, to forestall or overcome loneliness and boredom.

Prevention of alcoholism in the elderly may be approached through educational programs. The elderly whose world is constricted watch television and read newspapers or magazines which are excellent resources for education of the elderly and their families (33). It offers a wonderful opportunity to develop programs for family and friends concerning problems of aging, the need for support to the older person, and provides a medium to create a greater awareness to watch for signs in the older person who begins to drink too much. Treatment for older alcohol abuse patients consists mainly of group therapy, socialization and occasional antidepressants (34). Outcomes are as good or even better than with young alcoholics (31).

HAZARDS OF BED REST

As people grow older, they become less active and lead a more sedentary life. In nursing homes older people do less for themselves, particularly if the staff is impatient and would rather perform the activities of dressing and bathing for the patient rather than be bothered with the slowness or clumsiness of the resident. Helplessness is imposed upon the resident under the guise of helpfulness. Long hours are spent by the resident watching television or in sedentary group activities or taking naps and then back to bed. Mental and physical deterioration is predictable unless the elderly person has the initiative to remain active or unless energetic nurses or therapists provide encouragement and guidance. Prolonged bed rest predictably produces many complications (36, 37) (Figure 3.2). Muscles rapidly weaken and atrophy, osteoporosis develops, diminished endurance and fatigue ensue and mental functions wane. Prolonged bed rest results in contractures, particularly around the joints of the lower extremities. If these joints are not moved through the full range of motion when the patient is in bed, progressive limitation of motion develops. This is especially true in the case of the hip which is kept in partial flexion when lying on a bed, or sitting. A pillow under the knees increases flexion of the hip and maintains flexion of the

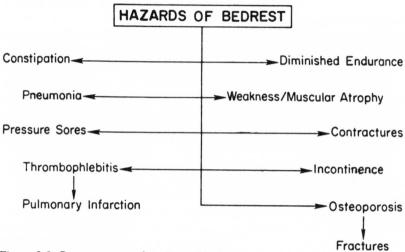

Figure 3.2. Consequences of prolonged bed rest.

knee. Both the hip and the knee must be fully extended for normal standing and walking otherwise greater muscular strength is required to support the body to prevent impairment of mobility. Maintenance of full range of motion of all joints is necessary. When a patient must support himself with incomplete extension of the hips or knees a greater muscular effort is required for standing and walking but also there is greater compression exerted on the joints increasing the wear and tear on joint surfaces and excessive pressure on bones.

Limitation of activity with bed rest produces progressive changes in the cardiovascular system. Even short periods such as 3 weeks of bed rest cause marked impairment of cardiovascular adaptability to the upright posture with an increase in pulse rate and a drop in blood pressure and sometimes the development of postural hypotension. This accounts for frequent dizziness, weakness and imbalance that is associated with ambulation after a period of prolonged bed rest. It sometimes requires 6 weeks or more to achieve full recompensation.

PREVENTION OF CANCER

The best method of cancer control is prevention. All health care personnel should engage in imparting reliable knowledge about prevention and management of cancer. Cigarette smoking has a carcinogenic effect and is implicated in causing lung cancer. There is an increasing incidence of lung cancer in women since smoking has become more popular in this group.

Screening of asymptomatic individuals for early detection of cancer is effective in eradicating cancer. The American Cancer Society has recommended guidelines for early detection of cancer and those that apply to the geriatric population are: Digital rectal examination every year, stool guaiac test for blood every year, sigmoidoscopy (flexible scope) every year for two years, then every 3 to 5 years thereafter for detection of colorectal cancer, pelvic examination every year, Papanicolaou test (PAP) two exams one year apart, then at least every 3 years for cancer of the cervix, breast physical examination every year and breast self-examination every month are recommended for screening for breast cancer (38). Mammography should be done annually in women who have a strong family or individual history of breast cancer. It is controversial whether annual mammograms are advisable for all women between 60 and 69 years of age (39).

Diet and nutrients are implicated in a causative role in the formation of cancer. Fiber from plants resistent to digestive enzymes possibly inhibit bowel cancer. Intake of fruits and vegetables, use of unrefined whole-grain products such as oats, wheat and rice are ingredients of a high fiber diet. There is some suggestion that increased cholesterol and bile acids enhance the risk of cancer and statistics indicate that endometrial cancer of the uterus and breast cancer correlate with obesity. There are other dietary components related to cancer that health professionals must be aware of as information becomes available.

REFERENCES

1. Glick, SM: Preventive Medicine in Geriatrics. *Med Clin N Amer, 60:* 1325, 1876.
2. Hazzard, WR: Preventive Gerontology: Strategies for Healthy Aging. *Postgrad Med, 74:*279, 1983.
3. Fletcher, DJ: Wellness: The Grand Tradition of Medicine. *Postgrad Med, 73:*87, 1983.
4. Treffert, DA: "Rustproofing" People: Wellness is Perspective. *Postgrad Med, 71:*179, 1982.
5. Shapiro, J; Shapiro, D: The Psychology of Responsibility. *N Engl J Med, 301:*211, 1979.

6. Cape, RDT: Nutrition and the Elderly. In *Fundamental of Geriatric Medicine*, Cape, TDT, Coe, RM and Rossman, I (Eds.). New York: Raven Press, 1983.

7. Baker, H: Hypovitaminosis in the Elderly. *Geriatr Med Today*, 2:61, 1983.

8. Schneider, CL; Nordlund, DJ: Prevalence of Vitamin and Mineral Supplement Use in the Elderly. *J Fam Pract, 17:*243, 1983.

9. Wooliscroft, JO: Megavitamins: Fact and fancy. *D M, 29:*1-56, 1983.

10. Schaumberg, H; Kaplan, J; Windebank, A, *et al.*: Sensory Neuropathy from Pyridoxine Abuse. *N Engl J Med, 309:*445, 1983.

11. Rosenberg, IH; Bowman, BB; Cooper, BA, *et al.*: Folate Nutrition in the Elderly. *Am J Clin Nutr, 36:*1060, 1982.

12. Shorvan, SD; Carney, MWP; Chanarin, I, *et al.*: The Neuropsychiatry of Megaloblastic Anemia. *Br Med J, 281:*1036, 1980.

13. Walsh, JR: Borderline Anemia in Old Age. *Geriatr Med Today*, 2:25, 1983.

14. Ghadirian, AM; Ananth, J; Engelsmann, F: Folic Acid Deficiency and Depression. *Psychosomatics, 21:*926, 1980.

15. Lynch, SR; Finch, CA; Mousen, ER, *et al.*: Iron Status of Elderly Americans. *Am J Clin Nutr, 36:*1032, 1982.

16. Disler, PB; Lynch, SR; Charlton, RW, *et al.*: The Effect of Tea on Iron Absorption. *Gut, 16:*193, 1975.

17. Walsh, JR, Cassel, CK; Madler, JJ: Iron Deficiency in the Elderly: It's Often Nondietary. *Geriatr, 36:*121, 1981.

18. Sandstead, HH; Henrikson, LK; Greger, JL, *et al.*: Zinc Nutriture in the Elderly in Relation to Taste Acuity, Immune Response and Wound Healing. *Am J Clin Nutr, 36:*1046, 1982.

19. Steffee, WP: Nutritional Intervention in Hospitalized Geriatric Patients. *Bull NY Acad Med, 56:*564, 1980.

20. Shaver, H; Loper, J; Lutes, R: Nutritional Status of Nursing Home Patients. *J Parent Enter Nutr, 4:*367, 1980.

21. Tomaiolo, P; Emman, S; Kraus, V: Preventing and Treating Malnutrition in the Elderly. *J Parent Enter Nutr, 5:*46, 1981.

22. Lipschitz, D: Protein Calorie Malnutrition in the Hospitalized Elderly. *Primary Care, 9:*531, 1982.

23. Pencharz, PB: Making a Nutritional Assessment. *Canad Med J, 127:* 823, 1982.

24. Blackburn, GL; Harvey, KB: Nutritional Assessment as a Routine in Clinical Medicine. *Postgrad Med, 71:*46, 1982.

25. Simon, HB: In *Sports Medicine*, Rubenstein, E and Federman, D (Eds.). Scientific Amer Med, NY 1983.

26. Sherin, K: Aerobic Exercise. *Postgrad Med, 73:*157, 1983.

27. Smith, EL; Gilligan, C: Physical Activity Prescription for the Older Adult. *Phy and Sport Med, 11:*91, 1983.

28. Hodgson, JL; Buskirk, ER: Physical Fitness and Age, with Emphasis on Cardiovascular Function in the Elderly. *J Am Geriatr Soc, 25:*385, 1977.

29. Morbidity and Mortality Weekly Report (MMWR) *USPHS, 30:*410, 1981.

30. Crossley, K; Irvine, P: Infectious Diseases and Immunizations. In *Geriatric Medicine*, Cassel, C and Walsh, J (Eds.). New York: Springer-Verlag, 1984, p. 311.

31. Atkinson, RM; Kofoed, LL: Alcohol and Drug Abuse in Old Age: A Clinical Perspective. *Substance Alc Actions/Misuse, 3:*353, 1982.

32. Bloom PJ: Alcoholism after Sixty. *AFP, 28:*111, 1983.

33. Brody, JA: Aging and Alcohol Abuse. *J Am Geriatr Soc, 30:*123, 1982.

34. Zimberg, S: Alcoholism in the Elderly: A Serious but Solvable Problem. *Postgrad Med, 74:*164, 1983.

35. Hartford, JT; Samorajcki, T: Alcoholism in the Geriatric Population. *J Am Geriatr Soc, 30:*18, 1982.

36. Asher, RA: The Dangers of Going to Bed. *Br Med J, 11:*967, 1947.

37. Kottke, FJ: The Effects of Limitation of Activity Upon the Human Body, *JAMA, 196:*117, 1966.

38. Guidelines for the Cancer-related Check-up: Recommendations and Rationale, *CA, 30:*194, 1980.

39. The Use of Diagnostic Tests for Screening and Evaluating Breast Lesions. Health and Policy Committee, American College of Physicians. *Am Inter Med, 103:*147-151, 1985.

CHAPTER 4

ASSESSMENT OF THE FRAIL ELDERLY

The following discussion will be a general framework of assessment referring only to some specific issues of care of the elderly and is not meant to be an exhaustive review of patient evaluation. For a detailed approach to the assessment of all people, the reader is referred to Caird's concise book (1). The goal of assessment is to gather relevant and useful information in a concise and efficient manner to identify client problems and needs and, thereby, prescribe care. There are important differences between old and young persons that health care providers must be aware of to gather optimal information. Some of the factors to be considered are: hidden disease, altered presentation of disease, multiple interacting problems, drug induced problems, the effect of environment on function, functional abilities, cognitive function, social supports, needs of the family and how to match the appropriate environment and services with needs. These factors are especially pertinent for the frail elderly when assessment occurs at critical times such as consideration for nursing home placement, or at a time of increasing dependency on family members.

Attitudes of some members of the health professions may negate appropriate assessment of the elderly. A feeling that therapeutic intervention is less relevant at this stage of life and that diagnostic or surgical procedures are unnecessary, predictably leads to a superficial examination. Similarly, a diagnosis of dementia may bias the examiner against the need for a good physical examination or preoccupation with psychosocial problems to the exclusion of medical needs can divert attention from a complete medical evaluation. To offset these negative influences, interdisciplinary assessment provides a balanced approach to influence decision–making in the management of older people.

A harmonious understanding between the examiner and patient leads to better data collection. Older patients may not be as alert or prompt in responding and the examiner must expect to spend additional time interviewing them. Techniques to promote a relaxed and informative interview with elderly people are listed in Table 4.1.

A patient's response during an interview may be influenced by either sensory or perceptual deprivation or by sensory overload which often influence cognitive ability, hearing and comprehension and performance in functional activities. Sensory deprivation occurs when activation of the sensory system is reduced, for example when a patient's room is isolated at the end of a hall, when a room has no windows or windows are beyond a client's visual field, when human contact is minimal, when radio, newspapers, or talking books are in short supply, or when clocks or calendars are absent. Conversely, sensory overload is the result of an excess in the amount or intensity of stimuli. For example, a patient may have up to six interviews upon admission to a health care facility, a television or radio may be playing in close proximity, there may be frequent distractions from paging over an

---

TABLE 4.1
TECHNIQUES TO PROMOTE EFFECTIVE INTERVIEWING

- When introducing each new assessment area, give the client time to process the "switch" before beginning questions.

- Monitor for overload (asking too many questions too quickly); give the client time to respond.

- If possible, conduct the assessment following a client's rest period.

- Conduct the assessment in a well-lighted room, limit window glare, avoid furniture that reflects light (glass, aluminum table tops).

- Ensure that the patient is using any corrective aids prescribed, e.g., glasses, hearing aids.

- Speak in a normal or slightly increased volume; do not shout. Lower the voice pitch, this is especially relevant for female interviewer. Face client with an unobstructed view of your mouth to facilitate lip reading.

- Speak slowly and distinctly, conduct the interview in a room with limited background noise. Avoid distracting noises such as rustling paper, tapping fingers, phone calls, chair movements, electric fans.

- Provide a comfortable room temperature. The room should be free of drafts. Drape client with bath blanket or sheet during physical examination.

intercommunication system, the client has undergone multiple therapies or activity programs and caregivers have changed frequently. Perception of sensory stimuli may be blunted or absent, occasioned by a decrease in patterning, meaning, or variability of stimuli. Other factors which influence perception include constant noise from an incorrectly placed hearing aid, room lights that are always turned on, or an environment which remains static with minimal changes in daily routines.

Disease is more common in the elderly and an elderly patient is likely to have more than one disease. Between three to seven chronic conditions have been uncovered in screening examinations of persons over age 65 with an average of 3.5 disabilities per person (2). Nursing home patients have been underdiagnosed, especially in ascertaining the cause of urinary incontinence, infections or the reason for falling.

Depression is common in the aged but must be differentiated from appropriate sadness related to the many losses incurred at this stage of life. The patient may experience sadness, apathy, worthlessness, have crying spells, feelings of guilt, difficulty in concentration and suicidal tendencies. However, thoughts of death and planning for burial are not uncommon in some elderly people and are not always a sign of depression. Anorexia and early morning awakening with difficulty sleeping are major features of depression. Many of the usual manifestations of depression may be missing in the elderly who may instead complain of abdominal or back pains, arthritic pain unrelieved by analgesics or multiple bodily complaints involving many organ systems, An elderly depressed person may become apathetic, withdrawn, uncooperative, unkempt and confused. A prior history of depression is helpful.

Falls are common in the elderly, however, reports of these occurrences are not often spontaneously volunteered by an older person. The clinician must specifically ask about falls. The patient frequently feels that this is just a part of aging. Since the incidence of falls is higher in the over 75 age group they occur at a time when there are also increased intellectual, neurological, sensory and physical impairments. The health care team must ascertain what the patient was doing at the time of the fall, whether consciousness was lost, how the fall occurred and how the patient recovered. Faintness occurring when arising from a chair or from a bed may suggest postural hypotension. A patient with nocturia who falls after arising from bed to go to the bathroom is typical of this condition. A feeling of faintness when looking up at a bookshelf or cupboard or when turning the head alerts the physician to a vertebrobasilar artery TIA, labyrinthitis or carotid sinus sensitivity. Patients who have arrhythmias may experience palpitations prior to a fall. Faintness or dizziness on exertion may be a symptom of aortic stenosis. Assessment for muscular weakness, gait disturbances, epilepsy, postural hypotension, cardiac dysrhythmia, aortic stenosis, are essential in a patient with a history of falls. In select patients, after other causes are excluded, carotid sinus sensitivity should be cautiously tested.

A particularly difficult group of patients to assess are those with memory deficits. Behavioral changes reported by the nursing home staff, spouse or other caregivers provide important clues to medical and mental problems. The onset of pneumonia, sepsis from pyelonephritis, subdural hematomas, and congestive heart failure may occur with changes in behavior. A health professional's long-term relationship and knowledge of the patient and their medications make subtle changes more obvious.

BASIC INTERVIEWING

Source and Reliability

Although there are circumstances in which it is advantageous to interview the patient and their spouse toegther, more often, unless the patient is comatose or has severe dementia, the patient should be interviewed alone. Even patients with diminished cognitive function may acurately describe symptoms. The health care professional may sometimes be unaware of the cognitive deficit until a mental status examination is done. To avoid being misled, a confirmatory interview with the caregiver, spouse, family, or a neighbor in the case of a patient who lives alone is necessary. When the patient is accompanied by a spouse or other relative, a courteous clinician may attempt to elicit the history with others in the room. This invariably leads to problems since the patient may defer to a spouse for answers or the spouse contradicts the patient which sometimes results in an argument or the patient withholds pertinent information to protect their privacy. It is usually better to interview them separately. Relatives or friends accompanying demented patients are sometimes uncomfortable talking in front of the patient, especially about issues of incontinence, wandering or other abnormal behavior. Likewise some patients are uneasy hearing others discuss their forgetfulness, incontinence or other problems.

Other information would be acquired from caregivers, nursing home staff or from old medical records whenever possible. Even mentally intact individuals may have misunderstandings of past diseases and treatment.

Chief Complaints

Multiple problems are typical of older people (2, 3) and accordingly the clinician should look for chief complaints rather than a single complaint. Actually, the main complaint of the patient may be found to be unimportant. Thus, incontinence, falls, shortness of breath, loss of weight and anorexia may be elicited only by direct questioning since the patient may consider that these problems are due to aging or is fearful because he/she perceives his/her complaints as serious illness.

The patient's complaint should never be ignored to address another problem with which the health professional is more concerned. What may bother a patient or the family may be different from what a health professional thinks are problems worthy of attention.

Habits such as smoking, drinking alcoholic beverages and drug use should be thoroughly explored. Alcohol abuse should not be assumed to be an illness of the young and middle aged. Recognition of alcoholism may explain previously undetected causes for confusion, falls and postural hypotension. Nutritional deficiencies are often a consequence of alcoholism.

Instead of the usual typical constellation of symptoms, an insidious slowly progressive decline may be the only manifestation of a physical or mental health problem. Disinterest in life, weight loss, agitated behavior can be subtle presentations for thyroid disease, chronic infections, malignancy, uremia, anemia, dementia, drug side effects, congestive heart failure, neurologic disease or depression. Concern about vague symptoms may come from a family member or neighbor rather than the patient who may deny that anything is wrong. Careful review of the duration and temporal relationship to other life events, i.e., the death of a loved one, a move from one residence to another, initiation of a new drug or a change in drug dosage, etc., may provide an answer.

Depression, anorexia, vague poorly characterized pain and confusion should not be dismissed as part of the aging process and consequently not worthy of evaluation. They may be caused by treatable conditions.

Hearing

Diminished hearing is obvious to family members and friends even if the patient is unaware of it. Some older people believe that using a hearing aid is a stigma associated with being old. The spouse or family often persuade the patient to obtain professional help. Hearing loss may invoke a paranoia in elderly people when the person hears sounds indistinctly or sees people talking and assumes that they are talking about him/her. Hearing loss restricts daily activities by preventing use of the telephone, listening to the radio or interacting with others at social gatherings.

Interviewers must be continuously aware of hearing problems. They should speak slowly and clearly, face the patient to provide visual clues and allow the patient to lip read. Speaking loudly or shouting often causes distortion by increasing the higher frequency sounds.

Cardiovascular

Shortness of breath (dyspnea), a common complaint of the elderly, most often indicates cardiovascular or pulmonary disease. Dyspnea associated with orthopnea (breathlessness when lying supine) are indicators of congestive heart failure. But dyspnea can be an anginal equivalent in older people, with shortness of breath overshadowing or replacing chest pain as a symptom of coronary insufficiency (4, 5). Weakness and confusion may be unusual symptoms of congestive heart failure occurring in the elderly. Similarly the clinical onset of myocardial infarction varies in the elderly. The older person may feel weak, faint or develop syncope instead of feeling chest pain. Painless myocardial infarction occurs with sufficient frequency to command attention of all health providers.

Edema, especially swelling of the legs, a common problem in the elderly is often due to congestive heart failure. However, edema from other causes is sometimes mistaken for congestive heart failure, consequently digoxin is often wrongly prescribed.

Peripheral edema of non-cardiac origin is due to chronic venous insufficiency, hypoproteinemia or due to sedentary habits.

Weakness, faintness, vertigo and syncope are frequent complaints of the elderly that often lead to falls. A common cause of these symptoms is postural hypotension. Normal asymptomatic elderly patients may demonstrate a decline of 20 mm mercury in systolic blood pressure when they stand.

Gastrointestinal

Anorexia may occur with infections, depression, dementia and from the effects of medication and, therefore, does not necessarily imply that gastrointestinal disease is present. Loss of appetite is a common and often perplexing symptom in the elderly.

Difficulty in swallowing (dysphagia) is another frequent and often confusing disorder in the elderly, often related to a neuromuscular problem or a gastrointestinal disease. An obstructive lesion ordinarily produces difficulty in swallowing solids initially but subsequently even with fluids. Conversely, difficulty in swallowing fluids initially implies a local neuromuscular problem or major neurological disease such as stroke.

Constipation is especially common in sedentary older people who lack bulk in their diets, have poor hydration, or from the effects of medication especially those with anticholinergic properties. Alternating diarrhea and constipation as in younger patients may be due to an underlying bowel carcinoma, or more likely in the elderly due to laxative abuse or a fecal impaction.

The stomach can hide large ulcers and tumor masses with a paucity of symptoms. Early symptoms of malignancy may be early satiety or weight loss, but may be dismissed by the elderly patient and/or relatives as part of the aging process.

Genitourinary

Frequency of urination and urinary incontinence are major causes of disability in the older person. Patients are too frequently referred to the urologist prior to obtaining adequate data and without performing an appropriate physical examination to exclude conditions that are correctable.

Older men may arise several times each night because of nocturnal frequency thereby causing loss of sleep for themselves and others in the household but more importantly it is also a time when injuries may be incurred from falling. When a patient has nocturnal frequency, inquiry should be made about the amount of fluid the patient ingests such as tea, coffee, beer and other fluids especially in the evening. Does the patient use a diuretic in the evening? If frequency is associated with burning and pain on urination, the possibility of urinary tract infection must be considered.

Incontinence of urine is a problem with multiple etiologies. It is particularly important to elicit the medications taken by the patient such as diuretics, anticholinergic preparations or sleeping pills. If the incontinence occurs during the hours of sleep it may well be that a sleeping pill has suppressed the cue to urinate. Elderly men with urinary frequency who subsequently develop incontinence may have the combined effect of bladder outlet obstruction from prostatic hypertrophy and overflow incontinence from the effect of an anticholinergic drug. A history of prostatic surgery in men may suggest that injury to the sphincter has occurred.

Inquiry should be made about loss of small amounts of urine when coughing, sneezing or laughing in women with a history of difficult childbirth and physical findings of a cystocoele or rectocoele and signs of vaginal estrogen deficiency. An urgent need to urinate with inability to get to the bathroom on time in a patient with dementia or residual neurological findings from a stroke makes the clinician attentive to urge incontinence. In addition to searching for precipitating factors and local urological problems, a neurological examination is important for the presence of an underlying lesion. Additionally, old people restrained in Geri–chairs or confined to beds with guardrails may have urinary incontinence because they are unable to get to the bathroom. This is a frequent cause in hospitals and nursing homes. The geographic distance of the bathroom from the patient's bed or chair may decide whether the patient is continent or incontinent.

It should not be assumed that the elderly are sexless and health professionals should be willing and interested in discussing sexuality and sexual problems. A question such as "Is your sexual life as fulfilling as you would like it?" indicates that the clinician is willing to discuss these problems if the patient so desires. Male impotence should engender questions about medication, diseases such as diabetes, recent surgery (Prostatectomy) or surgery for cancer of the colon with a new colostomy, or recent myocardial infarction. For the female patient lack of secretion due to atrophic vaginitis may be an important and treatable cause of dyspareunia.

Home Assessment

The evaluation of the elderly is not complete in many instances without a home visit by a member of the health care team or a community health worker to see how the patient will function in their environment or whether modifications are needed. Physical comforts, safety, heat, and cooking facilities should be evaluated. The home visit is an excellent opportunity to interview the caregiver of a chronically ill elderly person to assess their ability to cope with known problems and to identify potential problems which may not be obvious in other settings.

Social Networks

Social networks are important sources of help at times of crisis and stress and the health care provider should be knowledgeable of such support systems. Appropriate data should become an important element of the medical record and be recorded prior to any crisis. Social networks, both formal and informal, should be explored with the patient and his/her family as adjuncts to their available health care resources.

Financial Assessment

Many elderly live on fixed incomes which may limit their ability to secure appropriate health care resources. The expense of costly medication or laboratory and other diagnostic procedures could add considerable strain on an already limited budget. The health care provider should be aware of the financial abilities of their patients. However, decisions should be based on need rather than the ability to pay. Social workers provide an invaluable resource to aid the elderly person by sorting through eligibility programs so that they may obtain appropriate care. Alternative sources of funding such as insurance policies should be explored, and hidden community resources utilized.

Nutritional Assessment

The nutritional assessment begins with a dietary history and includes an exploration of dietary practices, medications, medical, psychological and socioeconomic factors that may influence adequate nutrition.

A nutritional history should include:
- Number of meals/day
- Type of food
- Weight change
- Appetite
- Difficulty in swallowing
- Dentures and ability to chew food
- Medications
- Alcohol consumption
- Exposure to sunlight
- Mental status
- Emotional status
- Marital status
- Meal preparation
- Cooking facilities
- Social connections
- Eating out
- "Meals on Wheels"
- Food storage (refrigerator)
- Transportation
- Cost of food
- Support system for shopping or cooking
- Physical disability

It is obvious that nutritional deficiencies stem from multiple factors, some medical but more often inadequate funds to purchase food, a disability that prevents shopping or cooking or the omission of meals due to forgetfulness. Depression is a common cause of loss of appetite in the elderly. Obviously problems differ if a patient is living alone, living with a spouse, or residing in an institution such as a nursing home or long-term care hospital. Visual or hearing impairments may produce difficulties in shopping. Absence of teeth may influence food selection. Physical problems such as a residual paralysis from a stroke, arthritis, or parkinsonism may interfere with cooking or the actual mechanical process of eating.

Clinical assessment includes documentation of weight change over a period of weeks or months, evidence of cachexia, muscle wasting, and skin fold thickness. It should be noted that measurements of skin fold thickness and arm circumference are somewhat limited by lack of standards for the elderly.

Preventive Measures

Nutritional habits should be evaluated. Women should be instructed to have breast examinations and should have a PAP smear. Patients should be asked about influenza and pneumococcal vaccinations and if tetanus immunizations have been renewed every ten years and if they are at risk for exposure to tetanus by working in the yard or garden.

Medications

A notorious cause of illness and disability in the elderly is an adverse reaction to medication. Any medications, but particularly new ones added to stable regimens should be immediately suspect when new symptoms develop. Not only are the elderly taking more medications than other age groups, but frequently apathy, mental confusion, and poor vision lead to medication errors. Prior to visits with a health care provider, the patient should be asked to bring in all medicines including over the counter drugs, thus allowing the interviewer to actually observe the number of medications being used. This simple procedure can often alleviate problems associated with poor memory, stress during the examination or ignorance of the patient about the actual type of medication being used. Home visits by the physician or a home health nurse should include a survey of medicines and method of administration.

PHYSICAL EXAMINATION

Much can be learned by observing patients walking into the examining room, sitting, standing and by their response during the interview.

Vital Signs

Blood pressure should be taken in both arms because of possible subclavian steal syndromes, but also should be taken lying, sitting and standing to elicit postural changes.

Temperature should be routinely measured. Autonomic nervous system dysfunction in old age is responsible for intolerance to heat and cold. The clinician must be constantly aware of hypothermia in winter and hyperthermia during hot summer weather. A low reading thermometer (rectal) should be available. If the thermometer reads below 35 degrees centigrade (95 degrees fahrenheit), low readings should be investigated and not simply attributed to thermometer malfunction.

Weight, a simple measurement which provides useful information for patient management, is often overlooked or not recorded. It is a measure of nutritional status, provides confirmation of weight gain or loss and is also useful to follow response to therapy such as diuretics.

It is useful to briefly describe the general appearance at the time of the examination including: State of nourishment, hydration or whether the patient is agitated or calm, cooperative or non-cooperative.

Skin

The skin of an elderly person becomes thin and dry and there is appreciable loss of elasticity in comparison to their younger counterpart. It is, therefore, difficult to use the skin to detect dehydration. An increase in capillary fragility is responsible for red to purple spots that appear usually on the hands and forearms (senile purpura).

Patients confined to bed or a wheelchair for long periods of time may develop decubitus ulcerations. There is a predilection over bony prominences which are subjected to pressure for extended periods of time such as heels, sacrum, scapulae, and occiput.

Hair

The clinician should look for the coarse tecture of hair characteristic of hypothyroidism. On the other hand, the loss of the outer one third of the eyebrow characteristic of hypothyroidism in younger age group is of less diagnostic value in the elderly person.

Eyes

Wrinkling and loosening of the skin around the eyelids produces extropian or eversion of the eyelids with exposure of the conjunctiva and often accompanying inflammation and tearing. On the other hand, entropian or incurving of the eyelids may produce irritation of the eyelids by the eye lashes. Tearing is decreased in the aged.

Vision

Visual acuity should be checked by use of the Snellen chart or, if practical, by reading a newspaper column. Check the person's peripheral vision. Each eye should be checked separately. Visual fields should be examined by the confrontation method. A careful ophthalmoscopic examination evaluates the cornea, lens and fundus. Some cataracts can be readily seen by inspection through the ophthalmoscope with 10 diopter magnification. Examination of the retina should be systematic and the optic disc should be carefully examined for papilledema, and changes due to glaucoma, the macula for evidence of macular degeneration and the fundi for evidence of diabetic or hypertensive retinopathy. Intraoccular tension may be measured with a tonometer.

Hearing

The ability to hear a watch tick with each ear or hear whispered voice sounds are gross estimates of hearing loss. The patient may have trouble hearing high frequency sounds that are similar. Audiometric studies are essential to document hearing losses and to determine losses at various frequencies.

The external auditory canal should be examined for wax (cerumen), pus or other discharges. Older persons with hearing losses should be evaluated for hearing aids. Health care providers should determine if hearing aids worn by patients are operational.

Cardiovascular Examination

Weight loss associated with anemia should be a signal to consider bacterial endocarditis. Fever may be absent in the elderly.

A firm to hard artery on palpation of the pulse is not clinically significant and is due to Monckeberg's medial sclerosis. The increased rigidity of the arterial wall causes a rapid upstroke in the pulse. Examination of the carotid arterial pulse for a delayed upstroke especially in the elderly patient with a systolic murmur suggests aortic stenosis. Additionally, an extremely rapid fall or collapsing pulse of aortic incompetence can be detected relatively easily.

Atrial fibrillation in the elderly should alert the clinician to consider thyrotoxicosis (thyroid hyperactivity) and pulmonary emboli. Every elderly patient with a recent onset of atrial fibrillation, an unexplained worsening of angina pectoris or congestive heart failure should be examined for hyperthyroidism.

Systolic murmurs occur in 60 to 80% of the elderly people, originating usually from the aortic area and are due to dilatation of the aortic annulus and ascending aorta, sclerosis or calcification of the aortic cusps. Aortic stenosis especially calcific aortic stenosis has a high incidence in the elderly and is distinguished by the characteristic systolic murmur at the base of the heart but sometimes even at the apical area of the heart, associated with a slow rising pulse of low volume (4). There may be mild clinically insignificant aortic regurgitation. Another form of left ventricular outflow obstruction found in the elderly causing systolic ejection murmurs namely hypertrophic obstructive cardiomyopathy (IHSS) is often misdiagnosed as aortic stenosis or mitral regurgitation.

Abdomen

An abdominal aortic aneurysm may be palpated on examination. However, a tortuous aorta can frequently be palpated in an elderly person and should not be mistaken for an aneurysm.

Acute appendicitis is relatively uncommon in the elderly and is likely to be overlooked. The pain may be poorly localized and peritoneal irritation may cause abdominal distention rather than abdominal rigidity (1).

Rectal Examination

Rectal examination provides invaluable information about the prostate in males, cervix and uterus in females, rectal wall and contents of the lower peritoneal cavity. Fecal impactions are detected and testing for occult blood in the stool may uncover lesions of the colon.

Genitourinary Examination

Women should have a pelvic examination for detection of cancer of the cervix and to monitor for endometrial cancer, especially if they are taking estrogen replacement therapy. Pap smears should be obtained. After two consecutive negative Pap smears one year apart rescreening is recommended every three years for women under age 60 but after this age no further screening is recommended (6). Obviously, clinical judgment should dictate the need for study at a more advanced age. Cervical cancer may be detected for the first time in an elderly woman especially those who have not had screening tests or who have not continued them (7). Postmenopausal bleeding or any unusual discharge should be investigated.

Neurological Assessment

Neurological disease often produces significant functional impairment in old age. An accurate functional assessment of older people with neurological disorders is crucial to determine appropriate rehabilitative measures and support systems.

Loss of frontal lobe inhibitory function produces primitive reflexes with abnormal facial and hand movements (primitive reflexes). The palmomental and glabellar reflex found in some normal old people is found more frequently in persons who have dementia. The palmomental is a contraction of the muscles of the lower chin when the thenar aspect of the palm is scratched. The snout reflex is formed by the lips pursing when the patient's upper lip is tapped with the finger and the suck reflex is positive if a sucking motion occurs when a straw or pencil is placed against the patient's lips. These primitive reflexes may be present in neurologically normal persons but if most or all of them are present in the same patient it usually supports evidence of cerebral pathology.

Absent ankle jerks and diminished vibratory perception in the ankle and foot are characteristic findings of the elderly (8). There is, however, controversy about such changes being strictly age related. Age related peripheral neuropathy itself is not clinically significant but may be meaningful when associated with visual, muscular or postural abnormalities. Clinically significant peripheral neuropathy suggests causes other than aging itself, such as diabetes, alcoholism and malignancy (9).

A systematic mental status examination is important in the examination of every elderly person. Critical functions tested include the level of consciousness, orientation, attention, expressive and receptive language, memory of immediate, recent and past events, constructional ability, and abstract verbal reasoning, mathematical, proverbs and statements requiring judgments. Occasionally a garrulous, older patient may appear to have normal mental capabilities, having learned to cope with intellectual impairment in a self-imposed gradually constricting environment. But a screening mental status examination uncovers obvious deficits. The cautious health care provider will not rely on global impressions but will perform a mental status examination. The short portable mental status questionnaire is a popular test that is effective in uncovering cognitive deficiency (10).

TABLE 4.2
SHORT PORTABLE MENTAL STATUS QUESTIONNAIRE
(SPMSQ)

1. What is the date today? _____
                                Month   Date   Year

2. What day of the week is it? _____

3. What is the name of this place? _____

4. What is your telephone number?_____
   a. (ASK ONLY IF SUBJECT DOES NOT HAVE A PHONE)
      What is your street address? _____

5. How old are you? _____

6. When were you born? _____
                                Month   Day   Year

7. Who is the president of the United States now? _____

8. Who was the president just before him?_____

9. What was your mother's maiden name?_____

10. Subtract 3 from 20 and keep subtracting 3 from each new number,
    all the way down.

SCORING: 0-2 wrong = Intact intellectual function
               3-4 wrong = Mildly impaired
               5-7 wrong = Moderately impaired
               8-10 wrong = Severely impaired

Allow one *more* error if only grade school education.
Allow one *less* error if education beyond high school.

FUNCTIONAL ASSESSMENT

Functional health represents the patient's ability to interact
with the environment. It depends on a combination of physical
abilities, mental activity, motivation and social influences
(environment and support network) (11). Unlike younger individuals, the elderly frequently develop conditions that lead to
lasting disability. Disability refers to the way that impairment
(pathologic changes) limits activities and functioning. Regardless
of the type or number of diseases or state of health, self-esteem,

autonomy and survival outside of the health care system depends on the aged person's ability for self-maintenance. Hence, it is important to evaluate the person's level of ability and activity, and often the patient's living environment to ascertain if the individual can function adequately or to see if the environment can be modified to meet the needs of the patient. A functional assessment should be part of every examination to determine effects of any physical and mental impairments and to decide what support systems may be needed. It is unwise to invest considerable time and expense on diagnostic and therapeutic procedures, while ignoring whether or not the patient can sustain therapy or even function in his or her environment.

A functional assessment itself does not predict where a patient should be placed. An assessment of the environment and support systems help to determine if a patient is able to cope with living in the community. Observing the patient in the home environment may be the key to successful discharge and long-term planning for some individuals with chronic conditions. For example, a stroke victim should not return home until availability of adaptive equipment and the persistence and motivation of the elderly person in becoming rehabilitated is evaluated.

A distinction must be made between some activities of daily living (ADL) which assesses bathing and grooming, dressing, toileting, eating, transfers, locomotion and the more complex instrumental activities of daily living (IADL) that may be necessary for independent living (11). The Barthel Index, Lawton's Physical Self-maintenance Scale and Katz's Index of ADL are examples of tools that can be used by health providers to assess ADL (12). The instrumental activities of daily living (IADL) measures the ability to use transportation, shop, cook, clean house, do laundry and use the telephone.

Items Used in Lawton's
Physical Self-maintenance Scale (ADL)

A. Toilet
   1. Cares for self at toilet completely, no incontinence.
   2. Needs to be reminded, needs help in cleaning self, or has a rare accident, weekly at most.
   3. Soiling or wetting while asleep more than once a week.
   4. Soiling or wetting while awake more than once a week.
   5. No control of bowels or bladder.

B. Feeding
    1. Eats without assistance.
    2. Eats with minor assistance at meal times, with special preparation of food, or in cleaning up after meals.
    3. Feeds self with moderate assistance and is untidy.
    4. Requires extensive assistance for all meals.
    5. Does not feed self at all and resists efforts of others to feed him.
C. Dressing
    1. Dresses, undresses, and selects clothes from own wardrobe.
    2. Dresses and undresses self with minor assistance.
    3. Needs moderate assistance in dressing or selection of clothes.
    4. Needs major assistance in dressing, but cooperates with efforts of others to help.
    5. Completely unable to dress self and resists efforts of others to help.
D. Grooming (neatness, hair, nails, hands, face, clothing)
    1. Always neatly dressed, well groomed, without assistance.
    2. Grooms self adequately with occasional minor assistance, e.g., shaving.
    3. Needs moderate and regular assistance or supervision with grooming.
    4. Needs total grooming care but can remain well-groomed after help from others.
    5. Actively negates all efforts of others to maintain grooming.
E. Physical Ambulation
    1. Goes about grounds or city.
    2. Ambulates within residence or about one block distance.
    3. Ambulates with assistance of (check one):
        a. ( ) another person
        b. ( ) railing
        c. ( ) cane
        d. ( ) walker
        e. ( ) wheelchair
            1) ( ) gets in and out without help
            2) ( ) needs help getting in and out
    4. Sits unsupported in chair or wheelchair, but cannot propel self without help.
    5. Bedridden more than half the time.
F. Bathing
    1. Bathes self without help (tub, shower, or sponge bath).

2. Bathes self with help in getting in and out of tub.
3. Washes face and hands only, but cannot bathe remainder of body.
4. Does not wash self, but is cooperative with those who bathe him.
5. Does not try to wash self and resists efforts of others to keep him clean.

Items Used in Instrumental Activities of Daily Living Scale (IADL)

A. Ability to Use Telephone
   1. Operates telephone on own initiative; looks up and dials telephone numbers, etc.
   2. Dials a few well-known telephone numbers.
   3. Answers telephone but does not dial.
   4. Does not use telephone at all.
B. Shopping
   1. Takes care of all shopping needs independently.
   2. Shops independently for small purchases.
   3. Needs to be accompanied on any shopping trip.
   4. Completely unable to shop.
C. Food Preparation
   1. Plans, prepares, and serves adequate meals independently.
   2. Prepares adequate meals if supplied with ingredients.
   3. Heats and serves prepared meals, or prepares meals but does not maintain adequate diet.
   4. Needs to have meals prepared and served.
D. Housekeeping
   1. Maintains house alone or with occasional assistance (e.g., "heavy work - domestic help").
   2. Performs light daily tasks such as dishwashing, bed making.
   3. Performs light daily tasks but cannot maintain acceptable level of cleanliness.
   4. Needs help with all home maintenance tasks.
   5. Does not participate in any housekeeping tasks.

The reader is referred to other sources for scoring and interpretation. Selection is not based on a preference of one instrument over the other but merely to indicate one method of assessment. Obviously there are more refined assessment instruments for research purposes but they are too unwieldy for everyday use in most clinical facilities.

Basic Laboratory

Laboratory tests are usually guided by the patient's problems, ability to cooperate and limitations of therapy imposed by invalidism of the patient. It is of little value to test for problems for which there is no intent to treat because of far advanced irresolute condition of the patient. On the other hand, there are conditions such as anemia, electrolyte disturbances, and infections to name a few, where treatment may substantially improve even seriously impaired patients. For routine examination a complete blood count, serum creatinine, electrolyte panel, and urinalysis suffice for most asymptomatic patients. Thyroid function should be assessed in older people with cognitive, cardiac and neurological disorders, even in asymptomatic patients. A stool guiaic for detection of blood in the stool should be a part of every initial physical examination and in the evaluation of anemia. Chest x-rays and electrocardiograms should be ordered for patients with symptoms or at risk of disease for example patients with a history of smoking, or a history of lung cancer, or a history of a malignancy known to metastasize to the lungs. Electrocardiograms should be ordered at appropriate intervals in patients with pacemakers, conduction disturbances, and histories of severe angina.

REFERENCES

1. Caird, FI; Judge, TG: *Assessment of the Elderly Patient*, 2nd Ed. Philadelphia, PA: J.B. Lippincott Co., 1979.

2. Williamson, J; Stokoe, IH; Gray, S, *et al.*: Old People at Home: Their Unreported Needs. *Lancet, 1:*1117, 1964.

3. Hodkinson, HM: *Common Symptoms of Disease in the Elderly*. 2nd Ed. London, England: Blackwell Scientific Publishing, 1980.

4. Noble, RJ; Rothbaum, DA: History and Physical Examination. In *Geriatric Cardiology*, Noble, RJ and Rothbaum, DA (Eds.). Philadelphia, PA: FA Davis, 1981, pp. 55-64.

5. Tinker, GM: Clinical Presentations of Myocardial Infarction in the Elderly. *Age and Aging, 10:*237, 1981.

6. Henderson, MM: PAP Smears. Current Recommendations on Their Frequency. *Consultant*, Jan. 1982, p. 77.

7. Kirk, EP: Gynecological Problems in the Elderly Woman. In *Geriatric Medicine*, Cassel, C and Walsh, J (Eds.). New York: Springer-Verlag, 1984.

8. Caird, FI: Examination of the Nervous System. In *Neurological Disorders in the Elderly*, Caird, FI (Ed.). Wright PSG, 1982, pp. 44-57

9. Huang, CY: Peripheral Neuropathy in the Elderly: A Clinical and Electrophysiologic Study. *J Am Geriatr Soc*, 29:49, 1981.

10. Pfeiffer, E: A Short Portable Mental Status Questionnaire for the Assessment of Organic Brain Deficit in Elderly Patients. *J Am Geriatr Soc*, 23:433, 1975.

11. Kane, RA: Instruments to Assess Functional Status. In *Geriatric Medicine: Fundamentals of Geriatric Care*, Vol. II, Cassel, C and Walsh, J (Eds.). New York: Springer-Verlag, 1984, pp. 130-140.

12. Kane, RA: *Assessing the Elderly: A Practical Guide of Measurement*. Lexington, Massachusetts: Lexington Books, 1981.

CHAPTER 5

REHABILITATION PRINCIPLES

Rehabilitation Medicine is the restoration of functional skills (physical, mental and social), which are a consequence of loss of function due to disability. For the frail elderly the challenge is to maintain ability to perform activities of self-care. The ability to meet one's own needs and retain bodily functions are a great concern to an older person.

Disability results from impairment in a person's capacity for mobility, communication, and social interaction (1). Loss of mobility occurs with pain, limitation of movement, deformity, weakness and instability, disorders of movement, sensory loss, loss of a body part such as an amputation, and from diminished exercise tolerance. Communication disabilities occur because of impairments of language, speech or voice use. Social interactions are compromised by cognitive deficiency, social deprivation, personality defects and inability to function in the community (1).

The goal of rehabilitation is to diminish disability by maximizing a patient's remaining abilities by progressively increasing their level of independence in activities of daily living. Appropriate planning for rehabilitation requires a thorough assessment of underlying diseases and disabilities, assessment of mental status and functional abilities relating to mobility, communication and social functioning (2), and the relation of the elderly person to his/her living environment. This is best accomplished by thorough medical and mental evaluation by the clinician, assessment of performance in functional ability and daily living such as the ability to communicate, feed, dress, bathe, move and toilet oneself and appraisal of the environment to assess social interaction. It must be stressed that rehabilitation medicine applies not only to the function of muscles and joints but should be used in the broader sense to include medical, physical, mental and psychosocial factors. For 60% of non-institutionalized adults over 85 years of age, functional impairments are consequences of heart disease, arthritis, visual and hearing problems, falls, cognitive impairment and drug reactions. The presence of multiple disease coupled with the age-related diminished reserve capacity of all organs influence the rehabilitation potential of the frail elderly. For instance, severe shortness of breath from advanced heart or pulmonary disease may hinder efforts to strengthen a patient with disabilities from severe arthritis or a stroke and will largely determine whether the patient will be able to remain at home or will need greater support or assistance in a nursing home. Fortunately for the patient with multiple disorders even small gains may be enough to improve functional ability sufficiently to allow a higher level of independence.

Rehabilitation is often viewed as a set of skills and procedures that nurses and therapists do rather than as a philosophy and total environmental approach to care. To be successful, emphasis should be on ability, a positive approach, rather than on disability (Figure 5.1). Even in a long-term care facility that emphasizes rehabilitation, verbal and non-verbal communications by staff often reward dependency of the elderly person instead of independent behaviors. Thus, the patient who washes his own face is less likely to receive encouragement than the person who is washed by the aide or the nurse. Overworked staff often reward dependency and disability as they spend time touching, talking and caring for the patient who cannot meet his own physical needs. Conversely, an elderly individual struggling to dress himself is either left unattended or is met by a busy caregiver who rushes to finish the task so that the patient will not be late for his/her therapy. It is paradoxical that these are the behaviors that we sometimes attempt to correct in family members who are overly helpful to an elderly person instead of urging him/her to be more self-reliant.

Appropriate rehabilitative goals for the frail elderly must be realistic and sufficient time must be allowed for them to be achieved. The initial step is the setting of goals with the patient and family with support and advice provided by members of the interdisciplinary team. The following examples demonstrate this process. For the frail elderly patient there may be limitations in the home environment, and their spouse may have his or her own functional limitations, chronic diseases or limited energy reserves. Thus, the expectation of returning an older patient to the care of family members even under supervision may be unrealistic. A

Elderly Person with Functional Limitations

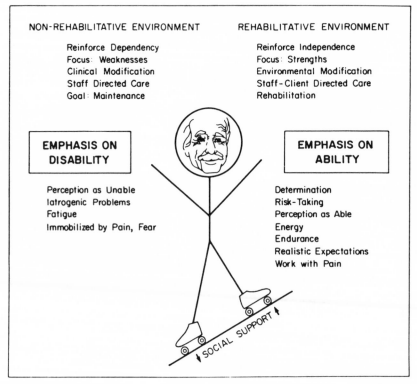

NON-REHABILITATIVE ENVIRONMENT   REHABILITATIVE ENVIRONMENT

Reinforce Dependency   Reinforce Independence
Focus: Weaknesses   Focus: Strengths
Clinical Modification   Environmental Modification
Staff Directed Care   Staff-Client Directed Care
Goal: Maintenance   Rehabilitation

EMPHASIS ON DISABILITY   **EMPHASIS ON ABILITY**

Perception as Unable   Determination
Iatrogenic Problems   Risk-Taking
Fatigue   Perception as Able
Immobilized by Pain, Fear   Energy
                                            Endurance
                                            Realistic Expectations
                                            Work with Pain

SOCIAL SUPPORT

Figure 5.1. Rehabilitation is more successful in an environment that fosters self-reliance. Poor results occur in an environment that reinforces dependency and helplessness.

more realistic goal must be defined, perhaps looking at another alternative level of care. However, if there is adequate community support a patient with the same degree of disability may be able to return home and thus achieve greater independence. Sometimes returning home may not be a desired goal held by either the older person or family. Problems with safety in the home, poor financial resources or self-neglect may be examples of chronic conditions that interdict return to home. Likewise, a socially isolated person may not wish to return to the home where he or she lived alone. On the other hand, contrary to an older person's desire to return home this goal may not be shared by the family or staff. This may be related to serious hazards in the home environment, inability of the patient to take care of himself because of inadequate support services or the family may have exhausted their resources in caregiving both physically and financially and see institutional placement as the only reasonable goal.

For the frail elderly person entering a long-term care facility such as a nursing home, there is a great need for rehabilitation, which may be contrary to the feelings of some health professionals and relatives who view it as a final place of residence. The goal of preparing the elderly person for maximum functioning, comfort, and security in an unfamiliar environment should be a focus for developing skills that will be encountered in that particular environment. Learning such environmental skills can be most important to their perceived comfort and well-being.

A major rehabilitation principle of the frail elderly is recognition of the process of thorough assessment of multiple interacting disease and disability. Rehabilitation is not an end unto itself, for example, a clinician must correct dehydration, electrolyte imbalances and problems of over-medication, treat infections, heart failure and other medical conditions that will have a bearing on rehabilitation. In addition, treatable causes of instability and falling should be evaluated and treated (1). If postural hypotension is present it should be corrected otherwise the patient will continue to fall. Pain must be controlled otherwise the patient may refuse to participate in therapy or treatment may be limited.

Early rehabilitation will avoid the deconditioning process that occurs with prolonged bedrest (1), and avoid concomitant weakness, fatigue, and shortness of breath that may dissuade the patient from participating in therapy. In addition, contractures and pressure sores are more likely to be prevented.

The use of both passive and active movement and exercise with assistive devices if necessary are important in caring for the elderly. A few examples of assistive devices are shown in Figures 5.2 and 5.3. Walking may be assisted by ambulatory support such as a walker or four-legged quadruped support. In a hospital or nursing home, even the stability offered by pushing a wheelchair may be helpful.

An increasing number of frail elderly people over the age of 85 are being referred for physical rehabilitation. A recent report has shown that well planned rehabilitation is effective in the very old patient and will return most people to their homes and they will show gains in such areas of self-care as feeding, dressing, bathing and continence and the ability to propel a wheelchair, to

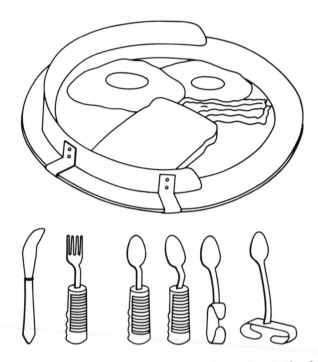

Figure 5.2. Adaptive eating devices: plate guards, rocker knife, fork and spoon for patients with hand disabilities.

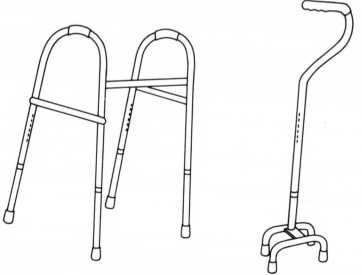

Figure 5.3. Ambulation aids: walker, quadruped cane.

walk or to climb stairs and to perform light housekeeping activities (3).

There are many factors contributing to poor results in rehabilitation. Among these are severe medical or physical impairment, inability to educate the patient, psychiatric problems, helplessness, an overly helpful caregiver, and poor motivation of the patient. Poor motivation of the patient is a problem to be solved rather than a reason to exclude a patient from therapy (4). Patients who are supposedly poorly motivated should be screened for medical and psychiatric conditions and particularly examined for cognitive dysfunction. Sometimes delirium needs to be resolved prior to a program for successful rehabilitation. Depression, common in elderly people is responsible for poor motivation. These patients should be treated with antidepressant drugs and should not be denied rehabilitation opportunities. Patients should be informed about the goals and the process of rehabilitation and the patient's strengths and weaknesses should be discussed. Caregivers may need to adjust their expectations of the geriatric patient who has experienced multiple losses. For some patients a more limited goal may be more realistic than that which the caregiver wishes.

Rehabilitation programs should not be restricted to the short time that a patient spends in the therapy unit or the time that a therapist spends at the bedside. It must be a continuous process to be most effective. A patient and caregiver must receive instruction to encourage continuation of the program on the hospital ward, in the home, or in the nursing home.

For the frail elderly, rehabilitation is a process concerned with improving the physical, mental, and psychosocial functioning of the patient while recognizing the interaction of disease, disability, and aging. Obviously this complex process of health care involves the expertise and skills of many disciplines if improvement in the patient's ability to function independently is to be achieved. The concept of the rehabilitation team is widely accepted. Typically the rehabilitation team is composed of physical and occupational therapists, physicians, nurses, social workers, psychologists and speech–language therapists. Each discipline contributes expertise from their professional domains which is used to assess, define, and implement the management plan. However, for the frail elderly the rehabilitative process is an on–going one involving many different disciplines whose needed expertise is defined by the needs of the patient.

Teamwork is a special form of interactional interdependence between health care providers who merge different but complimentary skills in the service of the patient and the solution of his/her health problem (1). Beckhard defines a team as "a group with a specific task or tasks, the accomplishment of which requires the interdependent and collaborative efforts of its members" (2). Even in its simplicity this definition is based on several assumptions:

1. The problem is so complex that it requires more than one set of skills or knowledge.
2. No one person can possess all of these skills or knowledge.
3. Forming a team of professionals with different skills will enhance the solution of the problem.
4. All members of the group are treated as equal possessors of relevant knowledge.
5. There is a common goal.

Thus, teamwork formalizes the process by which decisions are made and problems solved.

The relevancy to care of the aged is that the team approach enables health professionals to more easily define multiple problems and their potential interactions, to define reasonable goals and objectives and to identify available and appropriate resources. In some instances, the needs of the patient seem so overwhelming that no hope can be offered. However, this is one of the prime examples of a situation where the array of expertise offered by an interdisciplinary team can provide more creative problem–solving capabilities and thus improved patient outcomes.

Frequently, the solutions to complex health problems of the frail elderly do not lie within the purview of medicine, but instead may involve a wide variety of other health, community, and social services. It is, therefore, logical that the physician should not be expected to assume sole responsibility for all aspects of care or its coordination. The interdisciplinary team approach thus supports the concept that leadership is a function of expertise and changes based on the patients' needs and the knowledge and skills held by individual team members which are relevant to that specific need. However, it should never be assumed that all activities or tasks are carried out using a team. Teamwork is the process by which decisions are made and responsibilities are assigned. The team monitors itself through the process of establishing goals and objectives evaluating whether or not they have been accomplished.

There is no particular set of health professionals who must be members of the team. Composition of the team is defined by the needs of the population being served. One team structure which has recently emerged is the concept of the "core" and "extended" team. "Core" is defined as the team members who regularly function as a work group while the "extended" team is composed of individuals with whom the core team works closely on occasion (3, 4, 5).

Team members do not always have to work together, but one advantage of having team members in close physical proximity to one another is improved communication. Thus, the concept of team is actually a process whereby there is an integrated and coordinated effort toward problem solving or accomplishing tasks (6). It does not matter so much who the team members are, but instead emphasis is placed on whether the team is able to accomplish its objective.

For a team to be successful, it must follow a basic developmental process. First, the major step confronting a team is that of goal determination. If a team has no clear sense of its reason for being, it will not be able to determine its success. Secondly, roles and tasks must be defined. Professional roles and relationships vary depending on the organization and as staff changes it is often necessary to redefine the responsibilities of individual team members. Furthermore, the team members must also define the necessary tasks which need to be accomplished and assign them to various team members.

Thirdly, as the roles of various members change, i.e., the expanded role of the nurse practitioner, it may be necessary to re-examine the domain of professional practice and to assume new roles or to discard old familiar ones. This process of defining who does what is called role negotiation. Role negotiation is a necessary process if team members are to be utilized at their highest level of expertise and so that duplication of effort can be avoided.

In essence, a team must periodically examine its ability to work together and to provide an atmosphere which fosters cooperation and collaboration. Effective and efficient teamwork necessitates the following:

1. Common goals which are understood by all the team members.
2. Clear understanding by each team member of the role and its relationship to others in the team.
3. Clear understanding of the roles and relationships of other team members.

4. Mututal respect for and trust in other members of the team.

5. Effective methods of communication.

6. Periodic review of assessment of team functions.

In conclusion, teamwork is viewed as a process by which a group makes decisions and carries them out. However, just labeling a work group a team does not ensure teamwork.

REFERENCES

1. Hunt, TE: Practical consideration in the rehabilitation of the aged. *J Am Geriatr Soc, 28:*59, 1980.

2. Mayer NH: Evaluation. In *The Practice of Rehabilitation Medicine*, Kaplan, PE and Materson, RS (Eds.). Springfield, IL: Charles C. Thomas Publ., 1982, pp. 3-36.

3. Parry F: Physical Rehabilitation of the Old, Old Patient. *J Am Geriatr Soc, 31:*482, 1983.

4. Hesse, KA; Campion, EW: Motivating the Geriatric Patient for Rehabilitation. *J Am Geriatr Soc, 31:*586, 1983.

5. Baldwin, DC; Tsukuda, RA: Interprofessional Collaboration and Teamwork in the Care of Geriatric Patients. In *Geriatric Medicine: Fundamentals of Geriatric Care*, Vol. II, Cassel, C and Walsh, J (Eds.). New York: Springer-Verlag, 1984, pp. 421-435.

6. Beckhard, R: Organizational Issues in the Team Delivery of Comprehensive Health Care, *Millbank Mem Fund Quart, 50:*287-316, 1972.

7. Parker, AW: The Team Approach to Primary Health Care, Univ of California, Berkeley, 1972.

8. Andrus, H: The Health Care Team Concept and Reality. In *New Health Practitioners*, Fogarty International Series in Teaching of Preventive Medicine, Kane, RL (Ed.), (DHEW Pub. No 75-875), Washington, DC, 1975.

9. Lamberts, H; Riphagen, FE: Working Together in a Team for Primary Health Care — A Guide to Dangerous Country. *J Royall Coll Gen Prac, 25:* 745-752, 1975.

Part 2
COMMON PROBLEMS
OF OLD AGE

CHAPTER 6

DEMENTIA

Dementia must be differentiated from delirium. Delirium is characterized by disturbance of attention with fluctuating severity of impaired concentration, clouding of consciousness, and disorientation. There is often motor restlessness, somnolence, illusions and hallucinations. The symptoms occur abruptly and fluctuate considerably. It may occur postoperatively, associated with infections, cardiac, pulmonary, renal and hepatic failure, drugs and other medical disorders (1, 2). Delirium develops abruptly, is of short duration and non–progressive in contrast to dementia. It is often mistaken for dementia in frail older people who recover from delirium much slower than younger patients (3). Health providers must also be aware that delirium may be superimposed on an underlying dementia which is mistaken for worsening dementia (4).

Dementia, reaching almost epidemic proportions in the United States, will become an increasingly greater problem in the future because of the rapidly growing numbers of elderly people. The population over 75 years of age is escalating proportionately more rapidly than any other segment and by the year 2000 almost half of all the elderly will be over 75 years old. Additionally, the numbers of people 85 years old and older are increasing rapidly. Since dementia is primarily a disorder of old age these population characteristics are becoming more important. Presently it is estimated that the prevalence of a severe dementia is 4-5% (approximately 1 million persons) and that of mild to moderate dementia is 11-12% (approximately 3 million persons) (5). Dementia increases with advanced age being approximately 20% in persons over 80 years of age (6). It afflicts 58% of Americans in nursing homes (more than ½ million) (5). It is estimated that the lifetime risk of each of us alive today becoming severely demented may be as high as 20%.

At one time, dementia was considered to be due to cerebrovascular atherosclerosis found more prominently as people age. This viewpoint is no longer held. While the incidence of dementia increases with age, old age itself is not the cause. Studies have shown that 60 to 70% of dementias are senile dementia Alzheimer's type (SDAT) and that 15 to 25% are multiinfarct dementias (MID) and from 8–18% of dementia are mixed pathology (SDAT and MID) (5).

Alzheimer's disease (SDAT) sometimes mispronounced "Oldtimers disease" is a degenerative disease of brain cells with varying degrees of cerebral atrophy. The major pathologic changes are the presence of senile plaques, neurofibrillary tangles, and granulovacular bodies. The neurofibrillary tangles are found predominantly in the cerebral cortex especially in the hippocampus, the site of new learning. Chemical studies of the brain of patients with SDAT have shown a deficiency of acetylcholine and its enzymes choline acetyltransferase and acetylcholine esterase, enzymes that enhance and degrade acetylcholine respectively.

Clinical Picture

An elderly person with dementia shows a progressive decline in cognitive function that is variable from patient to patient. In addition to memory loss, the patient may show evidence of loss of judgment, inability to calculate, spatial disorientation, and personality change (irritable, irresponsible, withdrawn, mood swings). Dementia should be looked at as a spectrum of intellectual impairment from mild to severe. Too frequently, the term dementia is globally regarded as severe cognitive impairment and those with this diagnosis are stigmatized as being incompetent in all mental spheres. On the contrary, a demented person may be capable of making decisions regarding their personal life or give or refuse permission for surgical procedures even though they may need help with balancing their checkbook.

Usually, dementia is not difficult to diagnose. SDAT can be divided into three phases, the forgetfulness phase, confusional phase and dementia phase (5). In the earlier forgetfulness phase people's names or appointments are forgotten, there is difficulty remembering where things are placed (misplaced keys, money, bills, jewelry, etc.). The patient may write things down in order to remember them. Ordinary daily activities are not interfered with. During the second or confusional phase, memory for recent events is impaired, and orientation and concentration may be affected. Items from books or newspapers are not retained, there is difficulty finding words to express ideas, the patient may easily get lost, and there is difficulty coping with social activities. In the final dementia phase the patient is severely disoriented and mistakes the identity of spouse and friends, show marked memory loss and exhibit evidence of behavioral problems such as restlessness, delusion, hallucinations and paranoid thoughts.

Benign Forgetfulness

Some minor loss of memory in normal elderly people has been called benign senescent forgetfulness (7). This memory impairment is mild and not progressive in contrast to the more severe memory loss with dementia. Elderly people should not be concerned when they forget details of an event or a name since it is usually recalled at a later time.

It is often difficult to evaluate older persons with loss of memory for recent events since they often have less interest in current events. Memory impairment accompanied by anxiety, which is frequent among the elderly, may lead to a misdiagnosis of early dementia. Health providers must be cautious about overdiagnosis of dementia because of the attached stigma as well as the passive resigned attitude bordering on neglect by health professionals even for other associated disorders. Overdiagnosis occurs in equating cerebral atrophy on a CT scan with clinical dementia, mistaking depression for dementia, confusing expressive aphasia from a stroke with dementia, or failure to evaluate sensory losses (hearing, vision, etc.) any of which may give an initial impression of cognitive deficiency.

Diagnosis

The diagnosis of dementia is based on behavioral criteria since there are no chemical or physiological markers, that is, no laboratory or x-ray tests to assist in the diagnosis of SDAT. The diagnosis of SDAT is, therefore, made by excluding other causes of cognitive impairment. Therefore, all other conditions that produce dementia must be looked for to ascertain any cause that is responsive to specific treatment (3). Thyroid hormone deficiency (hypothyroidism), Vitamin B_{12} deficiency, brain tumor or blood clots, electrolyte or nutritional disorders, intoxications, infections or neoplastic disease must be considered as possible causes of either delirium or dementia or worsening an existing dementia. Therefore, a thorough examination that includes a complete medical, neurological, mental, and functional assessment, laboratory, x-ray and CT brain scan is indicated. The CT brain scan is valuable in diagnosing intracranial lesions such as brain tumor, or subdural hematoma. In SDAT, enlargement of the ventricles and cerebral atrophy are found on the CT scan. But these findings cannot be considered as specific for SDAT because similar changes are found in elderly people who show no obvious impairment of cognitive functioning and conversely CT scans of some severely demented patients may be considered within normal limits for their age.

Management

There is no drug that will cure SDAT. There are no effective treatments to reverse the course but rather the goal is to slow the rate of mental decline, improve the level of function and to remove factors (environmental, drugs, anemia, electrolyte disorders, etc.) that worsen dementia. Adequate management requires identification of treatable disorders that may precipitate or intensify the dementia. A demented patient has reduced brain reserve and even minor disorders may aggravate their mental condition giving an appearance of a more profound dementia than actually exists. Anemia, low blood sodium, dehydration, depression and infections are treatable and will improve both physical and mental state. Ascertaining the cause of fever and treating infections often mitigates the underlying dementia. Treating a depression may dramatically improve the patient. Many drugs may cause mental impairments that mimic dementia. Such drugs as tranquilizers (valium), sleeping pills, anticholinergic drugs (atropine-like psychosis), digoxin and diuretics are prominent in producing a delirium or aggravating a dementia. Visual and hearing impairments may lead to a misdiagnosis of dementia. The correction of sensory impairment by use of proper eye glasses, cataract surgery to improve vision, and hearing aids to correct hearing defects are often surprisingly effective in improving mental function and enhancing communication.

The goal in the management of senile dementia is to enable patients to remain at home and to foster attainable independence without exposing the patient to danger. A structured environment which provides consistent surroundings and predictable routine is necessary for demented patients (8) (Table 6.1). A characteristic of senile dementia is progressive deterioration of memory, intellect

TABLE 6.1
GUIDELINES FOR MANAGEMENT
OF IRREVERSIBLE DEMENTIA

• Treat reversible causes and associated medical conditions

• Maintain constant, predictable and familiar environment

• Schedule activities at same time each day — maintain a routine (arising, eating, medications, exercise)

• Make changes slowly, keep furniture in same place

• Keep familiar objects in sight (photographs, magazines, radio, TV)

• Use nightlights, calendars and clocks for orientation

• Keep patient ambulatory with daily exercise (walking)

• Avoid sensory overload (crowds, large spaces, complex conversations)

• Label rooms, sometimes with pictures or colors instead of words

• In early phases of memory loss use simple written instructions and reminder notes

• Refer to community agencies to help with patient and caregiver

and personality. Therefore, a patient becomes progressively more dependent on caregivers and family. Behavioral and emotional problems of a patient places extreme strain on the caregivers and family and may be factors for placement in a nursing home (9).

Health care providers must recognize that appropriate management of Alzheimer's disease includes not only treating the patient but offering guidance and support to caregivers who are trying to cope with the disease. This approach becomes increasingly important when the aim is to keep the patient in a home environment and independent as long as possible. The family must be educated about Alzheimer's disease and must become acquainted with those that can give support such as visiting nurse and social service agencies.

Help is available to families through the Alzheimer's Disease and Related Disorders Association which directs families to available resources in their area and provides educational material. Ten Basic Strategies for Families (Table 6.2) are recommended by the Society. *The 36-Hour Day*, a book which describes the realities of dementia, is another family guide (10). Health care providers must teach caregivers to cope with the anger, fatigue, depression, grief and frustration that occurs as the burden of care increases. The caregiver may become depressed or angry over the formidable

---

TABLE 6.2
TEN BASIC STRATEGIES FOR FAMILIES*

1. Obtain as accurate a diagnosis as possible; rule out all other causes; maintain a regular contact with a caring physician.

2. Realize and explain to others that Alzheimer's Disease *is* a disease and not insanity or stubborness; be open about the symptoms and progression.

3. Have a family meeting upon receiving the diagnosis; "hope for the best but plan for the worst;" an outside person might assist; all the family must be involved in the decisions and the care.

4. Work out all legal and financial issues that might arise, both the obvious ones and the hidden ones (even sticky money matters).

5. Strive to maintain the affected person's general health, level of activity, independence, and remaining skills as long as possible; use familiarity and routine to get through each day; go for long regular walks with the person; examine all safety issues (ID bracelet, double locks, reduced water temperature, etc.).

6. Focus on the needs of the primary caregiver also; develop a "cope notebook," line up emergency care; talk with others in the same situation, maintain health, both physical and emotional.

7. Carefully research resources for respite for primary caregiver and places when placement becomes necessary so these decisions are not made in crises.

8. If information seems difficult to find, keep trying, there is always someplace else that hasn't been checked.

9. Find a competent social worker or counselor for information and referral.

10. Above all, be as loving, patient, and objective as possible.

* *Developed by the Alzheimer's Disease Association to serve as a basis for recommendations.*

Used with permission from Alzheimer's Disease and Related Disorders Association.

---

modification of their own life due to the progressively heavier care that is needed for the demented patient (11). The spouse often must assume greater responsibilities and take on duties that they have never performed before; a wife may be required to handle financial matters and seek support for caring for her husband. Conversely, a husband with a demented spouse may be forced to undertake domestic work for which he is unfamiliar. As the disease progresses a spouse suffers more when communication skills of the demented person are lost, or when total care becomes an unremitting daily chore, when the patient wanders, keeps the spouse awake at night, or becomes incontinent. Respite care is an important consideration to allow rest for the caregiver. Day care programs offer respite for the caregiver while enabling the patient to remain at home for a longer time (12).

Sundowning or worsening of behavioral function after sunset is common in dementia. Confusion, restlessness, agitation and hallucinations occur at night possibly caused by loss of orienting cues associated with darkenss. A night–light and softly playing radio provides reassurance and orientation for some confused patients. Intensifying daytime activity sometimes may tire the patient and ensure more sleep at night. Small doses of antipsychotic medication such as thioridazene 10 to 50 mg or haloperidol 0.5 to 5 mg at bedtime may be helpful. Surprisingly good results sometimes occurs with lower doses.

Wandering behavior can make it impossible to care for the demented person at home or at day care centers. Wandering into busy street traffic, homes of strangers, or becoming lost in cold weather can be dangerous. Wandering often increases with any change of environment such as admission to a hospital or nursing home. Wandering is sometimes purposeful, the patient may be searching for her home or spouse. Wandering may occur at night which imposes greater strain on the caregiver. Demented patients who wander should wear identification bracelets, and/or carry an identification card with name, address and telephone number. Patients must be continuously reassured about their whereabouts and redirected to safer activities. Sometimes medications are necessary. Security measures may be necessary to protect the patient such as safety locks or latches, and child–proof doorknobs. Restraint of a patient in a gerichair or the use of Posey restraints often worsen the patient by increasing agitation and sometimes evoking hostile behavior. These measures should only be used as a last resort.

REFERENCES

1. Liston, EH: Delirium in the aged. *Psych Annals*, 8:49, 1978.

2. U'Ren, RC: Organic disorders in old age. In *Geriatric Medicine: Medical, Psychiatric and Pharmacologic Topics*, Vol. I, Cassel, C and Walsh, J (Eds.). New York: Springer-Verlag, 1984, pp. 553-576.

3. Small, GW; Jarvik, LF: The dementia syndrome. *Lancet*, 2:1443, 1982.

4. Reifler, BV; Larson, E; Hanley, R: Coexistence of cognitive impairment and depression in geriatric outpatients. *Am J Psych, 139:*623, 1982.

5. Schneck, MK; Reisberg, B; Fenis, SH: An overview of current concepts of Alzheimer's Disease. *Am J Psych, 139:*165, 1982.

6. Garland, PJ; Cross, PS: Epidemiology of psychopathology in old age: Some implications for clinical service. *Psych Clin N Am, 5:*11, 1982.

7. Kral, VA: Senescent forgetfulness: Benign and malignant. *Can Med Assoc J, 86:*257, 1962.

8. Rabins, P: Management of irreversible dementia. *Psychosomatics, 22:* 591, 1981.

9. Reisberg, B; Ferris, SH; DeLeon, MJ, *et al.*: The global deterioration scale for assessment of primary degenerative dementia. *Am J Psych, 139:* 1136, 1982.

10. Mace, NL; Rabins, PV: *The 36-Hour Day.* Baltimore, Maryland: The Johns Hopkins University Press, 1981.

11. Reisberg, B: Office management and treatment of primary degenerative dementia. *Psych Annals, 12:*631, 1982.

12. Fisk, AA: Management of Alzheimer's Disease. *Postgrad Med, 73:* 237, 1983.

CHAPTER 7

THE WET ELDERLY

Urinary incontinence, uncontrolled leakage of urine, is a significant and annoying problem to elderly people and their families. It strains family relationships when the family is unable or unwilling to provide care and it is frequently the final event that leads to placement in a nursing home. It often leads to embarrassment, isolation, and depression. The typical urine odor is offensive to visitors in the home or in a nursing home. Health professionals unfamiliar with incontinence are often responsible for inserting urinary catheters rather than first evaluating the cause of incontinence. After hospital admission, a wet bed is often a signal for insertion of an indwelling catheter, obviously for convenience of the staff, despite the absence of a history of incontinence prior to hospitalization. Physically or mentally impaired patients who have accidentally spilled their urinal have been wrongly labelled as incontinent. Health professionals are often uncomfortable with incontinent patients who must have other endearing qualities or exotic diseases to warrant adequate attention. The exact incidence is unknown but its prevalence increases with age. It affects 5 to 10% of elderly people in the community and greater than 25% of residents in nursing homes (1, 2). It is, therefore, a substantial drain on both human and financial resources.

In the process of aging, bladder capacity shrinks from 350–550 ml to approximately 250 ml. Associated with this diminished bladder capacity is an inability to retain large quantities of urine for normal lengths of time, resulting in frequency of urination. Normally, in adults awareness of bladder filling causes a nonurgent desire to void at about 250 ml but bladder contraction is normally inhibited by the central nervous system until voluntary micturition is initiated. In the elderly the urge to urinate may require hasty bladder emptying. If facilities are unavailable or too distant, incontinence may occur. In the frail elderly with diminished bladder capacity, continence is threatened by delay in finding or getting to the toilet due to poor vision or slower mobility or in situations where late cues to urinate require an ability to rapidly respond.

During bladder filling, stretch receptors in the detrusor muscle of the bladder are stimulated to pass impulses to the sacral spinal cord and when the bladder is full the impulse results in bladder contraction and urination (Figure 7.1.). Impulses from a higher brain stem center facilitates complete emptying. However, there is a cortical brain control which permits postponement of micturition. When the bladder is full, impulses from the sacral spinal cord results in an awareness of the urge to urinate. However, bladder contractions can be inhibited through impulses from the frontal cortex bladder center so that urination occurs at the desired time and place. Continence depends on an integrated

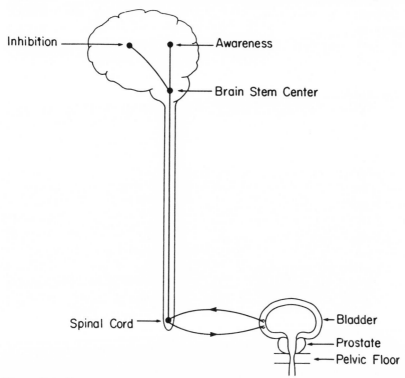

Figure 7.1. Central nervous system connections to the bladder showing reflex arc in sacral spinal cord with connections to the cortical awareness center in the parietal lobe and the inhibitory center in the frontal lobe which makes decision to either postpone or permit urination.

TABLE 7.1
PRECIPITATING OR AGGRAVATING FACTORS OF URINARY INCONTINENCE

FACTOR	EFFECT
DRUGS	
— Sedatives, hypnotics, alcohol	— Alter awareness of bladder cue
— Anticholinergics (antidepressants, antiparkinsonian)	— Urinary retention with overflow incontinence
DIURESIS	
Diuretics in pm, excessive fluids in pm, hyperglycemia, hypercalcemia	Frequency and loss of urine while in bed
ACUTE CONFUSIONAL STATE	
Drugs, acute illness, fever, dehydration	Decreased attention to bladder cues
URINARY TRACT INFECTIONS, ATROPHIC VAGINITIS	Irritable bladder with increased contractility
DEPRESSION/ISOLATION	Apathy with inattention to bladder cues
ENVIRONMENTAL	
— Unfamiliar environment, poor lighting, poor vision	— Difficulty locating bathroom
— Bed high, chairs too high and deep	— Decreased mobility → increased transit time
— Bed rails, chair restraints	— Unable to get to bathroom
— Bathroom facilities inadequate	
— Lack of privacy	— Disrupts normal pattern
— Toilet commode too distant	— Increased transit time
— Insufficient toilet aids (grab bar, elevated toilet seat)	— Person cannot position self for elimination
— Clothing inhibitors: restraints, buttons, tight garments	— Individual cannot get undressed
— Staff expectation of client incontinence: padding of beds, chairs, diapers	— Self-fulfilling prophecy

function of the bladder, urethra, pelvic floor and nervous system.

Incontinence in the elderly must be regarded as a symptom and not a diagnosis. It is often caused by a combination of decremental changes from aging and one or more of the factors shown in Tables 7.1 and 7.2. Incontinence should not automatically

TABLE 7.2
ESTABLISHED INCONTINENCE

Low Residual Urine	*High Residual Urine*
Urge Incontinence	Overflow Incontinence
(Detrussor hyperreflexia)	Hypotonic bladder
Urinary tract disorder	Bladder outlet obstruction
Cystitis	Prostatic enlargement
Urethritis	Urethral stricture
Prostatitis	Nervous system lesion
Vaginitis	Diabetes Mellitus
Bladder carcinoma	Pernicious anemia
Nervous system disorders	Tabes dorsalis
Uninhibited bladder con-	Tumor
tractions	
Dementia	
Stroke	
Spinal cord lesion	
Stress Incontinence	
Females — short urethra	
Pelvic muscle relaxation	

signal the need for a urological consultation nor should it elicit a defeatist attitude among health professionals. Approximately 50% of cases of incontinence are reversible and even a higher percentage is controllable. Incontinence is primarily due to dysfunction of the urinary bladder or its nervous system control.

There are several types of incontinence:

Urge Incontinence. Urge incontinence is involuntary urination due to an urgent desire to urinate that cannot be suppressed. Detrusor instability (hyperreflexia) occurs with any lesion which abolishes or suppresses the central nervous system inhibitory influence thereby allowing independent bladder muscle contraction. This is a common cause of incontinence, usually associated with stroke, dementia or Parkinsonism (Figure 7.1). Local bladder irritation from bladder infection can also trigger detrusor hyperirritability and result in incontinence. The patient gets an urge to urinate but is unable to get to the bathroom quickly enough to void.

Stress Incontinence. This type of incontinence is leakage of small amounts of urine with an increase in intraabdominal pressure from coughing, sneezing, laughing, running or lifting packages. It is most common in females and is caused by a loss of the angle between the bladder and urethra producing a funnel–shaped bladder outlet and shortened urethra (Figure 7.2B). Increases in intraabdominal pressure normally transmitted to the bladder and periurethral area are absorbed by the bladder and transmitted directly to the funnel–shaped urethra but not periurethrally (Figure 7.2B).

Overflow Incontinence. With bladder outlet obstruction from prostatic enlargement, urethral stricture or spinal cord lesions and peripheral neuropathies the bladder is no longer capable of normal contraction and emptying (Table 7.2). The bladder overfills and leaves an increased residual of urine in the bladder after voiding. The bladder eventually becomes large and overdistended. When the pressure in the overdistended bladder exceeds that exerted by the obstruction intermittent dribbling occurs.

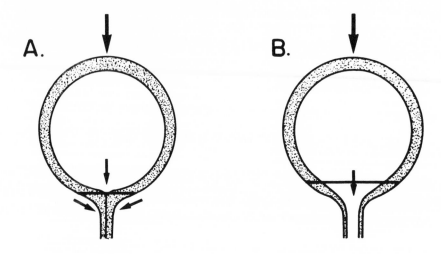

Women
  - • Weakened Pelvic Muscles
  - • Funnel - shaped Bladder Outlet
  - • Shortened Urethra

Figure 7.2. A) Normal Female Bladder. Increases in intraabdominal pressure produce an increase in pressure within the bladder and around the urethra. B) Weakened pelvic support structures cause intraabdominal pressure to be transmitted to the bladder directly to the funnel shaped urethra but not around the urethra. The result is stress incontinence.

Functional Incontinence. Due to limited mobility for example, from a stroke, arthritis, Parkinson's Disease or because of an unfamiliar environment, the patient is unable to reach the toilet in time to avoid an accident.

Iatrogenic Incontinence. Incontinence that results from medications, restraints or other physician induced problems.

Frequently there is more than one cause for incontinence. Often an elderly person initially able to cope with an underlying urological or nervous system disorder becomes incontinent when a precipitating factor (Table 7.1) is superimposed. A demented person with detrusor hyperreflexia may remain continent with a urinal, or bathroom facilities in close proximity, however, the administration of a sedative or tranquilizing drug may dull perception of bladder cues and thereby produce incontinence. A stroke or visually impaired patient in an unfamiliar environment may not find the bathroom quickly enough. An elderly male with bladder outlet obstruction from prostatic hypertrophy may develop overflow incontinence following administration of anticholinergic drugs. These drugs decrease detrusor muscle tone which makes the flaccid bladder capacity even larger and when superimposed on the bladder outlet obstruction overfilling of the bladder occurs.

EVALUATION

An adequate history detailing the factors listed in Table 7.1 and a thorough examination should elicit many of the causes of incontinence. A thorough data base addresses times and amounts voided, activities at time of incontinence, medications, awareness of need to void or defecate, bowel patterns and associated fluid intake. Often such a data base is not obtained because there is not consistent observation and documentation by all staff involved with the patient. Figure 7.3 is an example of a data base for urinary incontinence showing that the client was incontinent of a large amount of urine, without awareness, at 7:00 a.m. while lying in bed. Toileting at 8:00 a.m. had no results, but at 9:00 a.m. the patient voided 125 ml into the toilet at the staff person's direction. A post–void residual urine catheterization yielded 60 ml. A neurological examination and mental status evaluation is pertinent to demonstrate dementia, stroke, parkinsonism and other neuropathies. Abdominal palpation for an enlarged bladder, rectal examination for prostatic hypertrophy and fecal impaction,

FIGURE 7.3
DATA BASE — INCONTINENCE

TIME (Military)	ELIMINATION & AMOUNT X – Incont/Urine + – Incont/Stool Ⓧ – Cont/Urine ⊕ – Cont/Stool O – Toileted–No result R – Post-void Residual Catheterization	PT. REPORT A – Aware need to urinate/defecate NA – No report of need U – Urgency B – Burning, dysuria	ASSOCIATED ACTIVITIES A – Ambulation B – Lying in bed/sitting in chair T – Engaged in turning, E – Eating F – Dressing, bathing V – Visitors	FLUID INTAKE (cc)
0100				
0200				
0300				
0400				
0500				
0600				
0700	X – Lge. amt. in bed	NA	B	
0800	O		T, E	
0900	Ⓧ – 125; R – 60	NA		300
1000				
1100				
1200				

TOTAL EPISODES IN 24 HOURS:
Incontinence _____
Continence _____

TOTAL FLUID INTAKE: _____ cc

pelvic examination for atrophic vaginitis, and pelvic floor relaxation, laboratory tests for urinalysis, urine culture, vaginal cytology and a residual urine measurement are basic to assessing a patient with incontinence. Measurement of residual urine (catheterizing the bladder after the patient has urinated) is important prior to instituting any form of therapy and may be helpful in deciding which patients need further study by the urologist. Patients with increased residual urine will need further study for conditions shown in Table 7.2 and appropriate treatment given. Detrusor hyperirritability causing increased bladder contractions is one of the most common causes of incontinence and therefore empirical treatment with anticholinergic drugs or imipramine will often be successful even if no cause is found (3). Selected patients will need cystoscopic and further urinary tract studies.

MANAGEMENT

Frequently, an elderly person or family attempts to deal with the problem themselves and there is a delay in seeking health care until urinary incontinence has become a serious problem. An elderly person or caregiver limits fluid intake as a means of controlling incontinence which sometimes leads to dehydration and confusion. Frequent awakenings from wetness or urgency may cause poor concentration and sometimes confusion from lack of sleep. Urinary incontinence in a frail elderly person can cause skin excoriation and foster decubitus formation, the pain from which may inhibit transfer activities which interferes with bladder retraining programs. In an institutional setting, an incontinent individual often will be dismissed prematurely from an activity program or therapy session, either because of client embarrassment or staff reluctance to work with a wet patient. This creates problems from social isolation as well as limiting mobility gains from the programs. Thus, the health professional working with an elderly incontinent person must be prepared to deal with the consequences of the incontinence on mood, skin integrity, and mobility as well as with an individual and family who are frustrated and exhausted. The management of urinary incontinence, therefore, requires intensive effort and benefits from an interdisciplinary team approach.

From the data base a treatment plan is initiated (Table 7.3). Three approaches are recommended: maintenance of an inconti-

TABLE 7.3
SUMMARY OF APPROACH TO MANAGEMENT

• Correct or modify precipitating factors (Table 7.1)

• Enhance mobility and accessibility of toilet or urinal

• Use incontinence chart to record pattern of incontinence and to evaluate effects of bladder training and medication

• Institute bladder training program

• Anticholinergic drugs — to decrease detrussor muscle hyperirritability
        Propantheline (Pro-Banthine)
        Oxybutynin (Ditropan)
        Imipramine (also alpha–adrenergic agonist)

• Estrogen for atrophic vaginitis and urethritis

• Cholinergic agonist, Bethanechol (urecholine) for hypotonic (flaccid) bladder to stimulate detrusor muscle contractions

• Pessary and pelvic floor exercises for stress incontinence

• Surgery for — Stress incontinence
        Prostatic resection

• Incontinence underpants to absorb urine if penile clamps, condom catheters or surgical procedures are unsuccessful

• Long–term catheterization is a last resort

nence chart, alleviation of precipitating or aggravating factors of urinary incontinence (Table 7.1), and establishment of reasonable goals. A successful treatment plan for incontinence uses these three approaches in conjunction with interventions specific to the type of incontinence. An incontinence record shows the number of episodes, times, associated symptoms and activities and may provide clues to its cause and approach to treatment (4). Used properly, this record provides ready reference of improvement and serves as the basis for evaluation of the treatment regimen (5).

A major difficulty with the management of incontinence is failure of the client, family, or staff to see rapid improvement. One episode of incontinence with its attendant change of clothing or linen, quickly erases memory of the previous twelve hours of continence. Incontinence varies from mild to severe, thus the establishment of reasonable and meaningful short and long–term goals is critical to client and staff satisfaction. Bladder repatterning programs are unfortunately sometimes stopped after a few days because the elderly person continues to have episodes of incontinence, and the staff has ignored the record indicating a trend toward improvement. This unfortunately occurs when staff, family, and client fail to establish short-term goals.

SPECIFIC INTERVENTIONS

Urge Incontinence

Urge incontinence is a common type of incontinence frequently seen in institutions which care for the frail elderly with dementia and delirium. The treatment is often difficult to implement because of caregiver commitment required. Treatment consists of creating a positive environment, a bladder repatterning program, assurance of an adequate fluid intake, possible use of anticholinergic drugs (Probanthine, Ditropan, Imipramine) to decrease detrusor muscle hyperirritability, treatment of urinary tract infection and, with women, estrogen therapy for atrophic vaginitis and urethritis.

For individuals who have cognitive impairment, the staff must assume major responsibility in the bladder repatterning program. An elderly person is assisted to the bathroom fifteen to thirty minutes before the time when voiding previously occurred according to the bowel and bladder record. Generally the elderly person has a high degree of consistency with patterns of elimination. A review of the data base helps to refine the times of toileting as affected by activity, positioning, and fluid intake. Information about the number of incidents of incontinence or toileting with no results during the previous day is used to revise the schedule. With ongoing documentation and attentiveness to the elderly person's patterns, there is usually a marked reduction in the frequency of incontinence within two to three days.

Maintenance of an adequate fluid intake aids in reestablishing a normal pattern, provides adequate volume of urination and reduces bladder irritation. Dehydration among the frail elderly is not an uncommon occurrence. The individual with a cognitive impairment frequently has a decreased awareness of thirst and limited mobility and dexterity can impair access to fluids. In the institutional setting, a variety of between-meal and early-evening nourishments, such as juice, alcoholic beverages, sodas, fruit ices, gelatins, and soups can promote an adequate fluid intake. Often if fluid is limited following the evening meal, nocturia is reduced.

Again, the importance of a normal pattern of fluid intake and its relation to the timing of elimination must be emphasized.

Especially for an elderly person with cognitive impairment, the interaction between the patient and staff plays a major role in the control of incontinence. An older individual should be treated as an adult with the expectation of certain social behaviors, such as bladder control. Caregivers must impart a belief that the incontinence problem can be dealt with and that there will be an expectation of continence. Caregivers should be sensitive to communication which indicates dissatisfaction or frustration with the client when he is incontinent. Episodes of incontinence are dealt with quickly and quietly without chastising. Similarly, when an elderly adult is continent, praise is given in a quiet, adult manner relating to goal achievement and problem resolution.

The environment should promote general body and social awareness. A facility which is attentive to not only physical needs but also the social environment of patients is more likely to have success with a bladder repatterning program. By increasing total body awareness, a frail elderly person may become more sensitive to his internal signals, such as the need to void. The reestablishment of routines and functional ability are integral to the success of a bladder repatterning program. If possible, clients should be dressed in street clothes, including underwear. Other factors that may be detrimental to a bladder training program are use of a condom catheter because the older individual with memory impairment is unable to discriminate times and places when it is appropriate to be incontinent, i.e., when the condom is in place. Similarly the inappropriate overuse of the bedpan, urinal or bedside commode has the potential disadvantage of creating an unusual voiding location or position thus disrupting a retraining pattern. Conversely, if the individual urinates frequently at night or has marked pain with mobility these devices can be used at night with the person appropriately positioned. However, use of the bathroom is preferred because it provides privacy, behavioral cues, and reinforces normal physiological and behavioral patterns.

Implementation of a bladder repatterning program in a long–term care facility serving many frail elderly demented patients requires a team effort. A team approach supports staff by discussing incontinence problems, establishing reasonable institutional goals, implementing and evaluating the program, and airing frustrations. Through a team effort, a coordinated approach to bladder retraining can be promoted. For example, the activity directors and therapists may need to modify the schedule and duration of programs as well as to provide clothing and towels so that incontinent clients can be promptly assisted. Rather than scheduling patients activities around the bladder training program staff should be available to provide assistance during any scheduled activity, although in some instances it may be necessary to reschedule an activity according to the bladder program. The physical therapist may teach the patient transfer skills at the individual's toileting time. Dietary schedules could be examined in an effort to allow the nursing staff to assist clients to the bathroom prior to meals so that an elderly person would arrive unhurried at the dining room. Administrative support is reflected in personnel staffing and scheduling patterns, staff education and recruitment. The administrator who understands the importance of a bladder repatterning program may assist families and the community in understanding why they might occasionally find elderly residents to be wet.

An important aspect of a bladder retraining program is to promote continuity of a treatment regimen when a patient is discharged. The social worker fulfills this role by communicating this information to other health care agencies. An example of physician involvement is assessment and treatment of incontinence, eliminating its aggravating factors (Table 7.1) and in teaching other physicians to reduce the iatrogenic causes. Through a team approach, urinary incontinence can be managed successfully.

Stress Incontinence

A stepwise approach starting with medical management using imipramine and topical estrogen is advocated. From one-third to one-half of patients will respond to medical management alone. Surgical therapy is considered for medical failures. If the vaginal and bladder fascia have been overstretched and ruptured as a result of childbirth trauma or menopausal atrophy, surgery is usually indicated (1, 6, 7). Pessaries also are used with varying success in the treatment of cystoceles (1). To counteract the periurethral tissue atrophy, vaginal and oral estrogens are often used (8). Alpha-sympathetic agonists, such as phenylpropanolamine are effective drugs to increase intraurethral pressure and, therefore, urethral resistance to urine flow (2, 9). Imipramine, an antidepressant drug and sympathomimetic drugs also are showing positive results in the management of stress incontinence (10). Beta-adrenergic blocking agents, such as Inderal, also increases bladder outlet resistance.

Common interventions for the management of stress incontinence are exercises directed at strengthening the levator ani muscles which support the bladder and lower ends of the rectum and vagina (7, 8). For the elderly woman with stress incontinence, control of incontinence through exercise, toileting, and fluid-intake schedules may be a more desirable goal than the potential complete cessation of incontinence as a result of surgery. Modified Kegel exercises strengthen the pelvic musculature thereby increasing the function of the external bladder sphincter which reduces the amount of stress incontinence (8). Exercises should be fostered to strengthen abdominal muscles. Bladder emptying can be enhanced by abdominal tightening sometimes aided by hand pressure over the lower abdomen. Written and verbal instructions must be adjusted to a client's educational background and readiness to discuss the material.

The data base and bladder record are used to help the elderly client recognize peak times (e.g., upon arising) and events (e.g., laughing, sneezing) surrounding the stress incontinence. In this manner preventive toileting can occur and augment the benefits of the exercise regimen. Protective padding of undergarments may be necessary to reduce soilage and the associated embarrassment until pelvic muscles are strengthened. Numerous incontinence underpants are now available which need to be evaluated for cost, physical and emotional comfort, functional ease of application, cleaning and aeration to prevent skin maceration.

For elderly men, closely fitting cotton jockey shorts or a support strap can better accommodate a pad for occasional urinary incontinence. If external urinary sphincter tone does not return with an exercise regimen, then an external condom catheter may be necessary. Regardless of the external device or padding used, frequent skin inspection for areas of irritation is necessary. The perineal area should be cleansed gently with a soap and water solution and dried thoroughly at least daily. External urinary collection devices for females continue to be unsatisfactory.

Overflow Incontinence

Some elderly persons with overflow incontinence unrelated to bladder outlet obstruction, have decreased bladder contractions which may respond to cholinergic drugs such as Bethanecol chloride (11). Baclofen and dantrolene are medications used to relieve urinary retention resulting from detrusor-sphincter dyssynergy (9). Drug management has not yet shown consistent benefits among the elderly, but much investigation in this area is currently being undertaken.

Catheterization

Catheterization using either the clean intermittent technique or long-term indwelling catheterization are common methods of management for urinary retention with overflow incontinence. Although both methods of catheterization can prevent overdistention, the indwelling Foley catheter has been associated with almost 75% of acquired urinary tract infections in hospitalized patients (12).

There are advantages and disadvantages to each method. Intermittent self-clean catheterization gives the patient or caregiver control over the time of catheterization, freedom from drainage bags and catheters except at the times of catheterization, and allows participation in activities. The capacity for social and sexual expression is enhanced. The clean technique is dependent on handwashing and frequent catheterization to keep the bladder urine volume at less than 300 ml. It is inexpensive and can be performed anywhere that privacy is afforded. The clean–catheter technique uses a plastic or rubber catheter which can be reused and stored in a plastic bag. The catheter is rinsed with soap and water and flushed with water before and after use. Catheterizations are initially done every three hours, before sleep and upon awakening. The frequency of catheterization is reduced when residual urine decreases and is discontinued when residual volume is $\leq$ 100 ml (13). Residual urine is then measured once or twice a week for several weeks to assure that there is no worsening of bladder function. At times of voiding the help of lower abdominal pressure (Crede maneuver) aids in expressing urine from the bladder.

Intermittent catheterization is an effective method of bladder training as it allows for periodic emptying of the bladder without inhibiting contractions by the detrusor muscle as does an indwelling catheter (14). Thus, with retraining by regular toileting and increasing detrusor tone, which can be aided with medications, the frequency of catheterization often can be reduced and sometimes its need can be eliminated. It has also been an effective method to wean patients from indwelling catheters and subsequently freedom from catheter use (13).

Intermittent clean catheterization was developed initially with the goal of self-care for home management. If the patient is physically and mentally able, self catheterization is desirable. For an elderly person with cognitive impairment, it may be necessary for a spouse, relative or other caregiver to assume the responsibility. In hospitals and nursing homes, nurses or other health providers perform the catheterizations. As with indwelling catheterization, infections can be caused by poor technique and failure of the staff to wash their hands. Often, because of concern for the risk of infection, some hospitals and nursing homes will do intermittent sterile catheterization instead of the clean technique. This is more expensive, e.g., the need for sterile gloves and disposable catheters. Further study of costs, clean versus sterile technique, use of prophylactic antibiotics and staff performance are needed in long-term institutions.

Indwelling catheters are commonly used in hospitals and nursing homes for long-term catheterization but there is concern for the high incidence of urinary tract infections, kidney and bladder stones, urethral trauma, and the negative impact on the client's self-esteem and mobility. Leakage of urine around the catheter and discomfort is caused by detrusor irritability. This can be managed by anticholinergic drugs, such as Ditropan. Unfortunately, personnel often treat urinary leakage by inserting a larger catheter, which only serves to increase urethral and detrusor irritability. Indwelling catheters are appropriate to ensure comfort for seriously ill or terminal patients where frequent movement is painful, or by reducing skin breakdown of wounds and decubiti, and where trials of bladder retraining and drug management for incontinence have failed. Catheters need to be changed periodically because of encrusted material which consists of proteinaceous debris, calcium, phosphorus, magnesium, and uric acid, occurring more readily in an alkaline urine. Silicone catheters cause less encrustation than latex or Teflon catheters. Latex or Teflon catheters must be changed every three or four weeks whereas the silicone catheter will last from eight to twelve weeks. Acidification of the urine by administration of methenamine hippurate or ascorbic acid has been used to decrease encrustation and reduce the need for catheter changes. Methenamine is converted to formaldehyde which has an antibacterial action in the urine. However, a minimum of 60 to 90 minutes in acidic urine is necessary for conversion of methenamine to a high enough concentration of formaldehyde to be effective. It is clear that there is inadequate time for generation of formaldehyde in the urine of patients with an indwelling catheter and, therefore, it is of little value (13). Acidification of urine by oral intake of fluid, specifically cranberry juice, has been effective only when very large amounts of juice are ingested, which generally is not feasible for an elderly population.

Even with proper use of a closed, sterile indwelling catheter system for urinary drainage urine sterility is usually maintained less than two weeks (15). With the cumulative risk of infection, bacteriuria usually cannot be prevented for longer periods of catheterization. A higher incidence of bacteriuria has been associated with catheter and meatal cleaning and povidone–iodine solution (betadine) or soap and water than has occurred in patients who did not receive any cleaning regimen (16). To avoid introducing infection, urine specimens should be collected with a needle and syringe. To prevent urine reentry into the bladder the collection bag must always be kept below the level of the bladder.

Some patients have a history of long–term indwelling catheter use. Upon catheter removal, bladder urine retention may occur because of prolonged disuse of the bladder muscle (17). Reconditioning of the bladder prior to catheter removal, through catheter clamping and intermittent drainage, has been used commonly in the area of gynecology but infrequently in the care of the elderly. The catheter is clamped for three–hour periods, at the end of which it is unclamped for five minutes to allow complete emptying of the bladder. This cycle is repeated on three occasions prior to catheter removal. This technique results in earlier and more complete emptying of the bladder.

Not all patients with intractable incontinence require an indwelling catheter. Many male patients with an uninhibited bladder will require some form of condom catheter drainage for short–term use. Although appearing to be an innocuous procedure there are complications, e.g., penile edema, pressure erosions, skin irritation and maceration, and urinary tract infection (13). Adverse problems are more frequent with long–term use and in patients who are uncooperative usually because of dementia or delirium. These complications can be minimized by care in application of the condom, preventing accumulation of urine in the condom due to kinking of the tubing, and daily removal for washing and drying of the underlying skin. A condom catheter is not indicated for a distended atonic bladder; this is managed by inserting a catheter into the bladder.

REFERENCES

1. Williams, ME; Pannill, III, FC: Urinary Incontinence in the Elderly. *Ann Intern Med, 97:*895, 1982.

2. Ouslander, JG: Urinary Incontinence in the Elderly. *West J Med, 135:* 482, 1981.

3. Griffin, DJ: Urinary Incontinence in the Elderly. *Postgrad Med, 73:* 143, 1983.

4. Brocklehurst, JC: The Treatment of Incontinence. *Gerontol Clin, 9:* 298, 1967.

5. Clay, Elizabeth: Habit retraining. *Geriatr Nurs,* 1980. p. 252.

6. Kendall, AR; Stein, BS: Practical Approach to Stress Urinary Incontinence. *Geriatrics, 38:*69, 1983.

7. Mandelstam, Dorothy: Special techniques — strengthening pelvic floor muscles. *Geriatr Nurs, 69:*251, 1980.

8. Mohr, John, *et al.*:Stress Urinary Incontinence: A simple and practical approach to diagnosis and treatment. *J Am Geriatr Soc, 31:*476, 1983.

9. Williams, ME: A Critical Evaluation of the Assessment Technology for Urinary Continence in Older Persons. *J Am Geriatr Soc, 31:*657, 1983.

10. Rax, Shlomo: Pharmacological treatment of lower urinary tract dysfunction. *Urolog Clin N Am, 5:*323, 1978.

11. Applebaum, SM: Pharmacologic Agents in Micturition Disorders. *Urology, 16:*555, 1980.

12. Bielski, Michele: Preventing infection in the catheterized patient. *Nurs Clin N Am, 15:*703, 1980.

13. Warren, J; Muncie, HL; Berquist, EJ, *et al.*: Sequelae and Management of Urinary Infection in the Patient Requiring Chronic Catheterization. *J Urol, 125:*1, 1981.

14. Clean Intermittent Catheterization, CURN Project. JoAnne Horsley, Principal Investigator. San Francisco: Grune & Stratton, 1982.

15. Closed Urinary Drainage Systems, CURN Project. JoAnne Horsley, Principal Investigator, San Francisco: Grune & Stratton, 1981.

16. Burke, John, *et al.*: Prevention of catheter-associated urinary tract infections. *Am J Med, 70:*665, 1981.

17. Williamson, M: Reducing post-catheterization bladder dysfunction by reconditioning. *Nurs Research, 31:*28, 1982.

CHAPTER 8

BOWEL ELIMINATION PROBLEMS

Constipation occurs in up to 50% of people older than 60 years (1). Laxatives are, therefore, widely used at home, in hospitals, and nursing homes and it is estimated that between 15 and 30% of the population over 60 take laxatives regularly. There is a belief that a daily bowel movement is essential for good health, although studies have shown that many normal elderly persons have an evacuation only three times a week. There is no accepted number of normal bowel movements per week. Older people, therefore, are probably overly concerned about their bowel movements and the frail elderly particularly are apt to have fewer evacuations because of sedentary lifestyle, poor fluid intake, and dietary problems.

Constipation in the frail elderly is likely to be multifactorial (Table 8.1). The increased consumption of prepared, highly refined foods lacking sufficient fiber and bulk and an inadequate fluid intake are important factors contributing to elimination problems in the elderly. Food intake decreases with aging and loss of teeth and ease of preparation may lead to preference for soft, processed low bulk, high carbohydrate foods, which have little bulk and, therefore, slower intestinal passage. Conversely, the use of high fiber shortens intestinal transit time, produces larger stools, and more frequent bowel movements (2). Physical activity has a direct impact on large–bowel motility. Propulsive movement during and after food ingestion is rarely seen in the resting individual, but does occur in those who are physically active (3). Physical activity also aids indirectly in bowel function by maintaining tone in the support musculature of the abdomen and perineum. Decreased activity of the frail elderly related to functional impairment, combined with drinking too few fluids and eating a poor diet places this population at high risk for bowel elimination problems. Prolonged bed rest because of illness, weakness, or disability should be anticipated as a cause of constipation.

TABLE 8.1
MAJOR CAUSES OF CONSTIPATION

DRUGS
Anticholinergics
Aluminum-containing antacids
Opiates
Antihypertensives
Iron
Laxatives (chronic use)

ENVIRONMENTAL
Decreased physical activity
Decreased fluid intake
Low fiber diet
Barium GI x-ray studies

MECHANICAL OBSTRUCTION
Cancer
Inflammatory bowel lesions
Anal pain — Fissure / Stricture / Hemorrhoids

SYSTEMIC DISEASE
Depression
Dementia
Hypothyroidism
Hypercalcemia
Neuropathy

Drugs are an important cause of constipation and those listed in Table 8.1 are commonly used by the frail elderly (1, 4). Sometimes older people are taking two or three drugs that have anticholinergic effects. These drugs are notorious for developing constipation. Tricyclic antidepressants, antipsychotic drugs, some antiparkinsonian drugs have anticholinergic effects that decrease colonic muscular activity. Aluminum-containing antacids and barium sulfate used for gastrointestinal x-ray studies cause constipation by their physical properties in the bowel.

Overuse of enemas and laxatives produce serious consequences in regard to bowel function. It is estimated that between one in three and one in six individuals over the age of 60 takes at least a weekly dose of a laxative (5). In extended care facilities, laxatives are the single most frequently used class of drugs, with almost 60% of all patients receiving at least one daily (6). Prolonged use of laxatives eventually produces altered blood chemistries, with alternating diarrhea, a thin flabby colon, dehydration, and dependence for evacuation (7).

Constipation may cause symptoms of abdominal fullness (bloating), loss of appetite, headache, irritability, fatigue, a sense of depression, weight loss, and sometimes behavioral changes. Occasionally, more serious consequences occur (Figure 8.1). In the frail elderly person, symptoms may be mistaken for a severe systemic disease. Straining at stool produces deleterious effects on older people by reducing cerebral and coronary blood flow caused by the Valsalva maneuver. Hemorrhoids, and inguinal hernia may

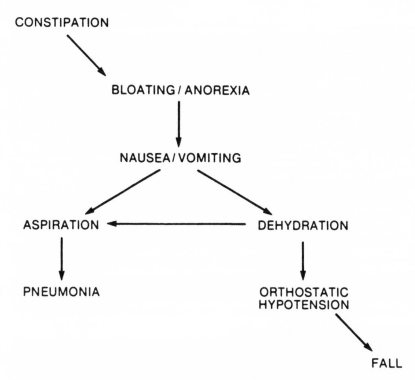

CONSTIPATION

BLOATING / ANOREXIA

NAUSEA / VOMITING

ASPIRATION ← DEHYDRATION

PNEUMONIA

ORTHOSTATIC
HYPOTENSION

FALL

Figure 8.1. Possible serious consequences of severe constipation or fecal impaction. (From P. Irvine, Patterns of Disease: The Challenge of Multiple Illnesses. In *Geriatric Medicine*, C. Cassel and J. Walsh (Eds.), 1984 with permission of Springer-Verlag Publishing.)

be worsened by straining at stool. Fecal impaction may additionally produce confusion, restlessness, tachycardia, vomiting and dehydration. A large fecal mass in the lower colon may compress the bladder and change the angle between the bladder and its outlet, the urethra, thereby causing either urinary retention or incontinence (1).

MANAGEMENT

Management of constipation involves evaluation for causes (Table 8.1) and includes a screening evaluation such as ditigal examination of the anus and rectum, and testing the stool for occult blood. A plain x-ray film of the abdomen can be helpful in determining the extent of fecal retention. The history and physical examination may quickly indicate the cause of constipation, but if not, or if there is accompanying weight loss, abdominal pain, or blood in the stool, a sigmoidoscopy and a barium enema may be necessary to evaluate the cause and suggest treatment.

A systematic record to monitor bowel elimination daily is helpful in determining the extent of the problem and the effect of therapeutic approaches. The addition of more fiber in the diet, introducing a routine exercise program, and drinking adequate fluids (1-2 quarts a day), and establishing regular toilet habits may adequately solve the problem of constipation. However, in frail elderly persons it may be necessary to add a laxative, suppository, or even an enema.

Dietary fiber, the undigested vegetable matter containing cellulose, hemicellulose, pectins, gums, alginates, and lignins, increase the size and wetness of stools by imbibing water to form a gel, and by osmotic effect of organic anions produced by bacterial action (2). Eating more fruits, vegetables, whole grain cereals and breads, dried fruits, will provide more fiber. The addition of unprocessed bran to cereals, fruits, or baked goods is a convenient way to increase fiber content of the diet. Several studies have shown that these dietary practices will increase spontaneous bowel movements and decrease the use of cathartics and enemas (8, 9). Sometimes it is not realistic to try to modify the roughage of diets by the above methods because of problems of

---

TABLE 8.2
TYPES OF LAXATIVES

BULK-FORMING AGENTS	LUBRICANTS
Bran	Mineral oil
Methylcellulose	
Psyllium	SURFACE-ACTIVE AGENTS
(Metamucil, Konsyl	Anthroquinone
Hydrocil)	cathartics
Polycarbophil	Cascara sagrada
Karaya gum	Senna
	Rhubarb
OSMOTIC AGENTS	Danthron
Magnesium salts	Castor oil
(Citrate hyroxide, sulfate)	Diphenylmethanes
Sodium phosphate	Biscodyl (Dulcolax)
Lactulose (chronulac)	Phenolphthalein (Ex-Lax)
Sorbitol	Docusate (Colace, Surfak)

dentition, anorexia, or difficulty swallowing in many frail, ill elderly patients.

A number of laxative preparations are shown in Table 8.2, and the choice for short-term use should be based on cost and potential side effects. An effective bowel program for the frail elderly patient is shown in Table 8.3 (8). The goal of repetition

---

TABLE 8.3
BOWEL PROGRAM FOR THE FRAIL ELDERLY

1. Assess patient for major causes of constipation.
2. If possible, discontinue drugs that cause or aggravate constipation.
3. After assessment, the following interventions may be required for severe constipation or impaction.
   a. Digital rectal manipulation to relieve impaction.
   b. Bisacodyl suppository administration if "a" is ineffective.
   c. Follow with a Fleet's enema if results are inadequate.
   d. Repeat process daily until constipation/impaction is resolved.
4. Provide instruction to the patient and family about the bowel program.
5. Fluid intake: Maintain a minimum of 1500 cc/24 hours fluid intake. Prune juice 4 oz (120 cc) is given with breakfast, and 4 oz (120 cc) of juice is served with lunch and dinner, daily.
6. The dietary program consists of 2 tablespoons of bran in hot cereal or All Bran cold cereal every morning. For variety, bran breads and muffins which have the same fiber content can be substituted.
7. Activity, exercise, and adequate food ingestion are encouraged.
8. LAXATIVE REGIMEN: Of several available regimens the following are two alternatives:

Alternative A
   a. Colace 100 mg once or twice daily
   b. Second day – Sorbitol 15-45 cc at bedtime if "a" is ineffective
   c. Third day – Biscodyl rectal suppository after breakfast if "b" is ineffective
   d. Fourth day – Fleet's enema if evacuation incomplete

Alternative B
   a. Biscodyl rectal suppository every other day in AM if no bowel movement the previous day. Toilet or commode fifteen to thirty minutes after suppository administration.
   b. Biscodyl tablet (5 mg) orally administered on the fourth evening if there has not been a complete evacuation during the previous four days.
   c. If still no results by day 5, a Fleet's enema is administered.
   d. The program is followed for an additional 5-day cycle. Should an enema be needed on day 10, then the amount of bran in the diet is gradually increased daily up to 4 tablespoons thereafter.

and patterning is that the individual will begin to respond to the bulk agents (bran and fluids) without the need for a suppository to stimulate the defecation reflex. However, there is no study to recommend one laxative over another. There are some clinicians who prefer osmotic agents over docusate (4). Lactulose is a synthetic carbohydrate which is not metabolized in the small bowel, but in the colon it is hydrolyzed by bacteria to osmotically active metabolites which hydrate the stool and increase reflex colonic contractions. Sorbitol 15–45cc administered at bedtime is less expensive and equally effective. Docusate (Colace), a stool softener appears to be effective in frail elderly patients despite a study that shows it to be ineffective for prophylactic use in the usual dosage (10). Obviously, further studies are needed to determine the most effective bowel program for frail elderly patients.

FECAL INCONTINENCE

Fecal incontinence is a significant problem that is not always acknowledged. In one study, fewer than half of the patients volunteered information about their problem with fecal incontinence (11). When fecal incontinence becomes a recurring issue in the care of the elderly, it usually becomes a deciding factor for nursing home placement. It is frequently due to remediable problems (Table 8.4) which should be the focus of assessment of this condition. In evaluating the patient, it is helpful to know if the stools are well formed or if they are loose, frequent stools. The latter are usually caused by fecal impaction, inflammatory bowel disease, diverticular disease, hyperthyroidism, autonomic neuropathy, or laxative and enema abuse, in addition to the factors shown in

```
┌─────────────────────────────────────────────────────────────────┐
│                          TABLE 8.4                                │
│                     FECAL INCONTINENCE                            │
│            PRECIPITATING OR AGGRAVATING FACTORS                   │
│                                                                   │
│      1. Fecal Impaction                                           │
│                                                                   │
│      2. Diarrhea                                                  │
│         a. Dietary (coffee, milk, fruit)                          │
│         b. Drugs (laxatives, antacids, antibiotics)               │
│         c. Environment (inaccessible toilet, bedrails, restraints)│
│         d. Immobility (stroke, arthritis, Parkinsonism)           │
│                                                                   │
│      3. Dementia and Delirium                                     │
└─────────────────────────────────────────────────────────────────┘
```

Table 8.4. Fecal incontinence with the passage of formed stools is encountered in patients with dementia due to an uninhibited gastrocolic reflex. It may occur with sedative drugs which dampen awareness, physical disability, and environmental factors which prevent getting to the toilet, and occasionally it is used by a patient to manipulate the response of caregivers.

The most common cause of fecal incontinence is an outgrowth from long–standing constipation (Table 8.1). Fecal impaction is a serious problem in the elderly that often causes diarrhea and fecal incontinence. It is easy to diagnose and is treatable. Feces above the impaction becomes liquified by bacterial action and liquid feces leak around the obstruction cuased by the hard impacted stool. A digital rectal examination will palpate the impacted stool if it is in the rectum. However, an impaction higher in the colon may be beyond the fingertip and can be detected by a plain x–ray of the abdomen.

MANAGEMENT

The initial approach is always to look for a correctable cause. A digital rectal examination and relief of the fecal impaction or constipation from any cause will often prevent fecal incontinence. Health care providers must anticipate factors that cause constipation and prevent it:

Immobility → Constipation → Impaction → Incontinence

Similarly, after a barium gastrointestinal study, the health care provider must remember that barium must be evacuated from the bowel. Diarrhea producing antacids or antibiotics are often overlooked as a cause of fecal incontinence. Drugs that diminish awareness of the need for a bowel movement must be eliminated. With demented patients who are unable to respond quickly enough to bowel cues, a bowel record can be kept. If formed stools are passed at predictable times, the patient can be placed on the toilet prior to the anticipated bowel movement. Retraining to establish a habit of bowel movements by taking advantage of a gastrocolic reflex after meals or fluids in the morning may be successful.

REFERENCES

1. Earnest, DL; MacGregor,   : Therapy for Gastrointestinal Disease. In *Drug Therapy for the Elderly*, Conrad, KA and Bressler, R (Eds.). St. Louis: C.V. Mosby, Co., 1982, pp. 189-196.

2. Almy, T: Fiber and the gut. *Am J Med, 71:*193-195, 1981.

3. Brocklehurst, J (Ed.): *Textbook of Geriatric Medicine and Gerontology,* 2nd Edition. London, England: Churchill Livingstone, 1978, pp. 369-370.

4. Elliot, DL; Watts, WJ; Girard, DE: Constipation: Mechanisms and management of a common clinical problem. *Postgrad Med, 74:*143-149, 1983.

5. Connell, AM, *et al.*: Variation of bowel habits in two populations. *Brit Med J, 11:*1093, 1965.

6. Lamy, P: *Prescribing for the Elderly.* Massachusetts: PSG Publishing Company, 1980, pp. 313-344.

7. Battle, E; Hanna, C: Evaluation of a dietary regimen for chronic constipation. *J Geront Nsg, 6:*527, 1980.

8. Miller, J: A nursing program for the management of bowel function in the hospitalized aged. *J Geront Nurs, 11:*37-41, 1985.

9. Sandman, PO, *et al.*: Treatment of constipation with high-bran bread in long-term care of severely demented elderly patients. *J Am Geriat Soc, 31(5):*289, 1983.

10. Goodman, J; Pang, J; Bessman, AN: Diotyl sodium sulfosuccinate: An ineffective prophylactic laxative. *J Chronic Dis, 29:*59, 1975.

11. Leigh, R; Turnberg, L: Fecal incontinence: The unvoiced symptom. *Lancet,* p. 1349, 1982.

CHAPTER 9

FALLS

Falling is common in old people with an increasing prevalence in the frail elderly. This progressive increase in falls ranges from 43% of women and 21% of men over age 65 (1) to 47% for women and 31% for men over age 80 (2). Women are not only more apt to fall but because of underlying osteoporosis they sustain more fractures. Over 8% of falls reportedly result in fractures (1, 2). Over 70% of fatal falls occur in people over age 65.

Accidents, clearly the most prevalent cause of falling in older people occur not only in people who are otherwise healthy but more often in those with an underlying disorder. Most accidents occur in or around the home which is not surprising since the frail elderly spend most of their time at home. Environmental hazards such as a poorly lighted staircase, loose scatter rugs, low tables, waxed floors and slippery bathtubs are especially dangerous for older people who have poor vision, unsteadiness, dizziness or other disabilities that predispose them to falls (3). The frail elderly fall more frequently because of dizziness, syncope, cardiac and neurological disease, general debility and functional impairment (Figure 9.1).

The incidence of falls is high in nursing homes because of a greater concentration of frail older people with physical disabilities and/or adverse effects of medication superimposed on diminished function of age (4). Most accidents occur when the patient is getting in and out of bed or wheelchair or getting on or off the toilet. Side rails on beds to protect patients may be responsible for a serious fall because a confused patient or a patient feeling the urge to go to the bathroom often attempts to climb over the bed rail. The alternative for the patient is to wet the bed and acquire the stigma of an incontinent patient. Personnel must be aware of these hazards. In nursing homes, residential homes, and hospitals environmental hazards should be removed, the texture of flooring, soles of shoes or slippers should be non–skid but on the other hand not too adhesive to impair walking for those patients who

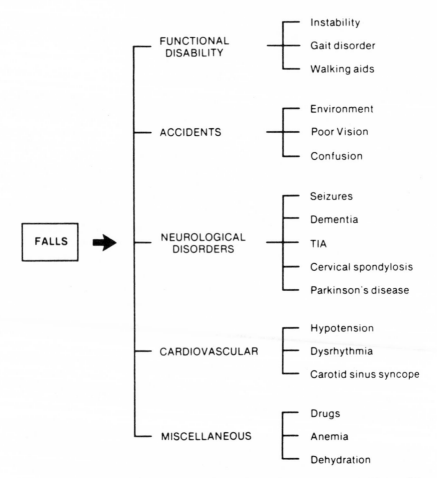

Figure 9.1. Major causes of falls. (From Walsh, JR; Bromberg, S; Miller, JG, *et al.*: Guidelines for Selected Geriatric Problems. In *Geriatric Medicine: Principles and Practice,* Cassel, C and Walsh J (Eds.). New York: Springer-Verlag, 1984, with permission of Springer-Verlag Publishing.)

have a shuffling gait. The design of bathrooms and toilets should be reviewed to minimize risks.

The cause of falls are usually multiple. Falling is predictable in patients with impaired function due to specific disorders (Figure 9.1). It is a serious mistake to treat the consequences of a fall and neglect correction of the underlying reason for falling. Falls occur as a result of either environmental factors, dysfunction of the patient or both (Figure 9.2).

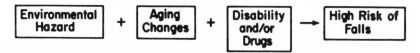

Figure 9.2. Risk factors in falls.

POSTURAL AND GAIT CHANGES WITH AGING

Standing depends on an intricate system of messages fed into the brain. Sensory input emanates from organs such as the eyes, ears (semicircular canals of the inner ear), and from position sensations of the head and neck, and lower extremities. Aging changes may reduce sensory input causing imbalance, unsteadiness, gait disturbances, and falling. Absent ankle tendon reflexes, loss of vibration and position sense, and slowing of maximal nerve conduction velocity in the lower legs, indicative of peripheral nerve degeneration are part of the aging process. Other postural and gait disturbances may increase the tendency to fall (5). The older person with a bent over posture who must extend the head to look upward and takes short shuffling steps is unstable when changing direction and is apt to fall. A shuffling gait often causes the frail older person to trip or stumble over seemingly minimal obstacles.

Since falls most often result from a combination of factors, the clinician should not be satisfied to discover a sole cause but should look further for associated conditions. Visual impairment which is common in the elderly is a major factor in causing falls especially when combined with other disabilities. Older frail people with poor vision from cataracts, macular degeneration and glaucoma associated with impairment of mobility from a neurologic or an arthritic disability will predictably have more falls than if they had normal vision. Visual perception of the vertical and horizontal which often worsens with aging may be a significant additive factor responsible for falls in a hemiplegic patient (6). Visual cues become increasingly important in patients with poor ankle and foot position sense. Similarly alcohol has a profound effect on a frail, impaired elderly person who may cope with their limitations until they drink alcohol. Many older people are hidden alcoholics and alcohol is probably responsible for more episodes of falling than realized. Orthostatic hypotension, cardiac arrhythmias, vestibular disease, medications and alcohol predispose to falls and should be evaluated in any patient with a history of repeated falls. Some specific causes for falls are described in this chapter and others shown in Figure 9.1 are discussed in other chapters.

SOME SPECIFIC CAUSES OF FALLS

Postural (Orthostatic Hypotension)

On standing, a drop in systolic blood pressure is a normal response. Ordinarily adaptive mechanisms protect blood flow to the brain by increasing blood return to the heart, and an acceleration of heart rate to maintain cardiac output. However, adjustments to postural change is slower in older people. Failure of the normal compensatory physiological mechanisms results in venous pooling of blood, causing reduced venous blood return to the heart and a diminished cardiac output, the consequences of which are poor cerebral perfusion and syncope. Syncope is a sudden temporary loss of consciousness due to lack of oxygen delivery to the brain.

The magnitude of the decrease in systolic blood pressure on assuming an erect posture is greater in older people. The range of fall in systolic blood pressure that establishes a diagnosis of postural hypotension is between 10–30 mm Hg. Yet a fall of 25 mm of mercury in systolic blood pressure is sometimes observed in asymptomatic older people. On the other hand, a decrease of 20 mm of mercury systolic pressure which produces symptoms is abnormal. Therefore, the critical diagnostic feature is the accompanying presence of symptoms with a drop in blood pressure. But, even a drop of 20 mm of mercury or more in an asymptomatic older person should alert the health care provider that there is a risk of precipitating symptoms with further exposure to factors predisposing to postural hypotension, e.g., medications (antidepressants, antihypertensives, nitrates), anemia, dehydration and prolonged bed rest. Members of the health care team should anticipate problems and take measures to prevent them.

Typical clinical features of hypotension are light headedness or faintness, blurring or loss of vision, weakness and unsteadiness, especially when arising from bed or from a chair. A classical scenario is an elderly man who gets out of bed because of nocturia, faints and falls because of postural hypotension. Confusion and urinary incontinence may occur. Instability of balance, syncope and falls with its consequences may start an unfortunate series of events that culminates in serious disability (Figure 9.3).

To establish the presence of postural hypotension, supine and standing blood pressure measurements are taken at intervals of one or two mintues for ten minutes. Some older people develop symptoms after walking for a few minutes so that measurement of the blood pressure after such exertion may be helpful to show the drop in blood pressure. Postural hypotension, a physical finding, is not a diagnosis and further evaluation is necessary to determine its cause. A careful history of drug intake, evaluation for significant fluid and blood loss, and study for adrenal abnormalities should be undertaken. Tachycardia accompanying postural hypotension is a helpful clinical clue. With volume depletion (dehydration) the autonomic system is intact, therefore, standing produces tachycardia whereas with autonomic nervous system dysfunction a concomitant increase in heart rate is lacking. Autonomic nervous system dysfunction is frequent in the frail elderly and, therefore, this compensatory mechanism may be blunted (7). It is relevant to reiterate that assessment of elderly individuals for postural hypotension even if asymptomatic is crucial before prescribing drugs which may aggravate the condition and thereby produce symptoms.

Symptoms from postural hypotension may be mollified by correcting the underlying disorder if possible. A prospective program should be initiated to minimize risks of falling by educating the patient, staff and family on preventive measures. Patients should be instructed to exercise the legs by flexing the feet and knees while supine in bed, sitting with legs dangling over the edge

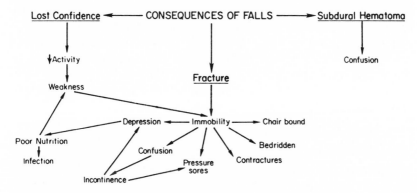

Figure 9.3. Serious consequences of falls.

of the bed for several minutes before standing up, clenching fists to increase heart rate, and using support stockings. Staff responsibility includes identifying and removing offending drugs, replacing fluids, treating anemia, and prescribing appropriate exercise during prolonged bed rest with early ambulation and occasionally cautious use of salt or salt–retaining hormone (fluorohydrocortisone).

A recent study showed significant reduction in systolic blood pressure associated with syncope within 35 minutes after starting to eat in nursing home patients (8). In addition, ten elderly patients had a decrease of blood pressure without syncopal episodes. There was no associated compensatory increase in the pulse rate in response to the drop in blood pressure. However, a blunted increase of pulse rate in response to a fall in blood pressure occurs in many healthy elderly subjects. The hypotensive response to eating was possibly due to splanchnic blood pooling or other local intestinal factors in patients with inadequate baroreflex compensation or a failure of sympathetic nervous system activation in response to insulin. These patients had multiple diseases which may have contributed to the hypotensive events. In evaluating falls, dizziness or syncope in older people this mechanism should be considered.

Carotid Sinus Hypersensitivity

Hyperactivity of the carotid sinus reflex is found in approximately one-third of older men with atherosclerotic and hypertensive heart disease. Stimulation of the carotid sinus in the neck may cause syncope or a transient clouding of consciousness without actual fainting. It is recognized, however, that a hyperactive carotid sinus is common in older people which most often is asymptomatic. Carotid sinus syncope occurs in only 5 to 20% of persons with a hyperactive reflex (9). Syncope from other causes may occur in an older person and the hyperactive carotid sinus reflex itself may not be responsible. Other causes should be sought prior to automatically treating the hyperactive carotid sinus.

Typically, the patient has syncope when hyperextending the neck during the process of looking upward at a high shelf or the sky, or turning the head when backing a motor vehicle, or with pressure on the neck from a collar, or with sneezing. Manual pressure over the carotid sinus produces a slowing of the pulse or a drop in blood pressure.

Mechanical stimulation of the neck produces vagal stimulation and consequently one of three responses in the patient with a hypersensitive carotid sinus (10). The most frequent response is to produce a slow heart rate (bradycardia). An infrequent response is lowering the blood pressure (hypotensive effect) without slowing the pulse. And thirdly, syncope may occur with both a low blood pressure and a low pulse rate, the so–called mixed response which is infrequent. Rarely carotid massage produces transient or even permanent neurologic deficits. The maneuver is, therefore, recommended only if other diagnostic studies for the cause of falls are not helpful (9).

A patient with an asymptomatic hyperactive carotid sinus does not need treatment. Avoid high collars for the few cases in which this is the precipitating factor. Therapy is required for repeated syncopal episodes or syncopal episodes that occur when driving. The most effective form of treatment is the insertion of a cardiac pacemaker (10). Large doses of anticholinergic drugs have been used to speed the heart rate, but are often poorly tolerated, particularly in older people, and may not abolish symptoms.

Other Cardiac Disorders

Arrhythmias may produce transient cerebral dysfunction, syncope and falls (9, 11) due to a decrease in cerebral circulation stemming from a reduced cardiac output or a reduced systemic blood pressure. Aortic stenosis causes syncope typically associated with exertion (7). The average life expectancy after the onset of syncope in patients with aortic stenosis is three years.

Drop Attacks

A drop attack is a sudden transient, unexpected loss of postural tone in the legs causing a fall but no loss of consciousness (12). Turning of the head or neck, looking upward toward the ceiling or sky sometimes precipitates the attack. The loss of muscle tone and strength in the legs causes difficulty in standing up again unless pressure is placed on the soles of the feet which seemingly provides postural orientation. Drop attacks have been implicated as a cause of approximately one-fourth of all falls. The event is usually considered to be related to brainstem ischemia from vertebrobasilar artery insufficiency due to either atherosclerosis or to external compression of the vertebral artery secondary to cervical spondylosis. Carotid sinus hypersensitivity may also produce a drop in blood pressure with brainstem ischemia and consequently a drop attack. Drop attacks may be produced by a number of disorders that cause transient reduction in vertobrobasilar artery blood flow. Therefore, in an elderly patient with atherosclerotic tortuous vessels, or cervical spondylitis, a superimposed anemia, postural hypotension, cardiac arrhythmia, carotid sinus hypersensitivity or hypoxia may precipitate a drop attack (12). Elimination of these precipitating factors may prevent drop attacks.

CERVICAL SPONDYLOSIS

In the frail elderly, cervical spondylosis (degenerative joint disease involving the cervical vertebrae) associated with tortuous arteriosclerotic vertebral arteries has been said to cause diminished blood supply to the brain on rotation and extension of the head. This seemingly plausible explanation has recently been challenged. Cervical spondylosis, a common disorder of elderly people leads to osteophyte formation and degenerative disc disease which sometimes produces narrowing of the spinal canal, compression of the spinal cord and nerve root by osteoarthritic changes encrouching on the intervertebral foramina. It becomes clinically significant when patients develop an aching neck, pains in the shoulder and arms, signs of sensory impairment, weakness, wasting of muscles and loss of reflexes in the upper extremities. Subsequently, motor and sensory changes appear in the lower extremities. The gait becomes slow and stiff-legged, tendon reflexes are increased and there is loss of position and vibratory sensations. With these neurological signs and symptoms, the finding of typical bony changes of the cervical vertebrae on x-ray suggests the diagnosis. However, correlation between bone changes on x-ray and neurological manifestations is poor. Many older people have advanced arthritic changes on x-ray but are asymptomatic. The demonstration of bony changes on x-ray alone is not sufficient evidence to explain falls. With significant neurological findings, injection of dye into the spinal canal (myelography) may show compression of the cord and interruption at vertebral discs.

Treatment of mild cases with a cervical collar may be sufficient. However, elderly people who experience progression of symptoms and more serious neurological impairments must have surgical decompression to arrest progress of the disease.

CONSEQUENCE OF FALLS

Most falls produce no clinical sequelae. Nonetheless, the high prevalence of falls with advancing age results in a large number of injuries. Consequences of falls are shown in Figure 9.3 and are serious. Fractures and subdural hematoma cause major morbidity and may even be responsible for deaths. Death rates from falls are less than 50 per 100,000 at age 65 and increase progressively to 525 per 100,000 over age 85.

Fracture: The most common consequence of falling is bony fracture. Even minor falls may produce a serious hip fracture in an older person. Underlying osteoporosis plays a large role in fractures (see Chapter 11).

A frequently overlooked outcome of repeated falls is the sequence of events that stems from a loss of confidence. Fear of falling results in withdrawal from activities, isolation and loneliness. Older people consider falls a result of aging and are reluctant to tell their doctor about them until a major traumatic insult occurs. Therefore, frail elderly people should be specifically questioned about falls.

Subdural Hematoma: Subdural hematoma may result from head injury but falls are so common in the elderly that the episode of trauma may seem inconsequential and not recalled by the patient. Sometimes there is no history of falls. Bleeding from veins in the subdural space is more likely to occur in individuals who have an enlarged subarachnoid space, increased vascularity and diminished supporting tissue allowing more mobility of the brain within the skull. Subdural hematoma is, therefore, more common in the elderly. It should be especially considered in the alcoholic, patients undergoing dialysis treatment for renal failure, or treatment with anticoagulants.

The hematoma may develop to considerable size over days or weeks before producing symptoms. Chronic headache may be the only symptom especially associated with coughing, sneezing or straining at stool. The diagnosis of subdural hematoma must be considered in the very elderly patient who develops intellectual deterioration such as delirium, dementia or with a sudden worsening of an existing dementia. Symptoms result from general pressure on the brain rather than focal brain damage. Personality change within a few months of the fall, clouding of consciousness or coma without hemiplegia or hemianopsia suggests subdural hematoma. Nurses, aides or family may be the first to observe bizarre behavior patterns. Fluctuating neurological signs and symptoms, considered to be characteristic are found in only about a third of the cases. Skull x–rays, CT and radionuclide scans are useful diagnostic measures. A neurological consultation should be obtained early.

Other Complications

Burns may result from falling against a stove or fireplace, hypothermia may ensue if surrounding temperature is low, dehydration can also occur if there is prolonged delay in discovery of the victim of a fall. As shown in Figure 9.3, confusion, pressure sores, depression, and incontinence are sequelae to falls that can be anticipated and often prevented.

MANAGEMENT OF FALLS

Clearly, the management of falls is an interdisciplinary task (Table 9.1). Most falls are accidental and preventive measures should be undertaken to eliminate hazards in and around the home and in nursing homes. Obstacles should be removed to avoid tripping and floors should be maintained with non–skid surfaces. Highly polished slippery or wet floors are dangerous to frail

---

TABLE 9.1
MANAGEMENT OF FALLS

- Evaluate and treat specific cause
- Remove environmental hazards
- *Build confidence — remove fear of falling*
- Exercise legs in bed before arising
- Clench fists to increase heart rate
- Rehabilitation to strengthen muscles, use assistive devices, correct or modify gait and posture
- Remove offending drugs
- Replace body fluids
- Support stockings
- Careful use of salt–retaining steroids
- Cervical collar for drop attacks

oldsters with shuffling gaits or precarious balance. Adequate lighting is necessary especially for those who have nocturia and visit the bathroom frequently. Older people must be taught that it is dangerous to quickly rise from bed to a standing position. A few moments of flexing the feet and the legs will improve venous return to the heart, sitting up and dangling the feet over the edge of the bed for a few minutes allows postural adjustment prior to standing. Episodes of postural hypotension may be averted by these simple maneuvers. Strengthening of muscles, particularly leg muscles, teaching the patient with poor balance to turn in a semi-circle instead of abruptly turning or using canes or walkers to assist in maintaining balance are effective measures to prevent falls. Old people who have repeated falls should be taught how to get up after falling. An effective program will give the patient more confidence to cope with disability and prevent withdrawal from meaningful activities.

REFERENCES

1. Sheldon, JH: *The Social Medicine of Old Age.* London: Oxford University Press, 1948, pp. 96-105.

2. Exton-Smith, AN: Clinical Manifestations, In *Care of the Elderly. Meeting the Challenge of Dependency*, Exton-Smith, AN and Evans, G (Eds.). London: Academic Press, 1977.

3. Walsh, JR; Bromberg, S; Miller, JG, *et al.*: Guidelines for Selected Geriatric Problems. In *Geriatric Medicine: Principles and Practices*, Cassel, C and Walsh, J (Eds.). New York: Springer-Verlag, 1984.

4. Kalchthaler, T; Bascon, RA; Quinton, V: Falls in the Institutionalized Elderly. *J Am Geriatr Soc, 26:*424, 1978.

5. Sabin, T: Biologic Aspects of Falls and Mobility Limitations in the Elderly. *J Am Geriatr Soc, 30:*51, 1982.

6. Tobis, JS; Nayak, L; Hoehler, F: Visual Perception of Verticality and Horizontability Among Elderly Fallers. *Arch Phys Med Rehabil, 62:*619, 1981.

7. Lipsitz, LA: Syncope in the Elderly. *Ann Intern Med, 99:*92, 1983.

8. Lipsitz, LA; Nyquist, P; Wei, JY; Rowe, JW: Postprandial Reduction in Blood Pressure in the Elderly. *N Engl J Med, 309:*81, 1983.

9. Kapoor, WN; Martin, D; Karpf, M: Syncope in the Elderly: A Pragmatic Approach. *Geriatrics, 38:*46, 1983.

10. Walter, PF; Crawley, IS; Dorney, ER: Carotid Sinus Hypersensitivity and Syncope. *Am J Cardiol, 42:*396, 1978.

11. Gordon, M; Huang, M; Gryfe, CI: An Evaluation of Falls, Syncope, and Dizziness by Prolonged Ambulatory Cardiographic Monitoring in a Geriatric Institutional Setting. *J Am Geriatr Soc, 30:*6, 1982.

12. Lipsitz, LA: The Drop Attack: A Common Geriatric Symptom. *J Am Geriatr Soc, 31:*617, 1983.

13. Rowe, JW: Falls. In *Health and Disease in Old Age*, Rose, JW and Besdine, RW (Eds.). Boston: Little, Brown Co., 1982.

CHAPTER 10

PRESSURE SORES

Decubitus ulcers, also called pressure sores and sometimes bedsores are areas of skin breakdown where prolonged pressure has deprived the area of adequate blood circulation. The inadequate blood flow through the capillary bed within the skin results in tissue necrosis. Pressure sores develop in the home, acute hospital care setting and in nursing homes. Pressure sores develop in 8.8% of hospitalized and home care patients and approximately 70% of patients with pressure sores are over age 70 (1). Pressure sores may develop within two week of hospitalization, which parallels the time of greatest immobility and reinforces the need for early preventive action.

Frail elderly patients are at risk for pressure sores. The risk is increased for patients who are bedridden or confined to a wheelchair because of a neurological disorder, advanced illness, coma, dementia, or arthritis and in patients with bowel and bladder incontinence (2, 3). Other factors that may contribute are malnutrition, protein deficiency, anemia, peripheral vascular disease and oversedation. Moisture from perspiration or incontinence macerates the skin and incontinence particularly is considered to be one of the more important predisposing factors for pressure sore formation (4). Elderly persons with loss of sensation and immobility from stroke, peripheral neuropathy, dementia and oversedation are at risk. A loss of the protective response of pain sensation and a paucity of position shifts enhance the risk. Frail elderly people with atrophic skin, loss of subcutaneous fat and loose skin folds lose the cushion effect over bony prominences and are subject to shearing forces on the skin. Shearing forces over the sacral area are frequently created by a partial sitting position in a cranked-up hospital bed or any position that allows a sliding effect of the body's weight on the loose skin. The amount of pressure on the skin of the buttock of an elderly person seated on two inches of foam padding in a wheelchair far exceeds the normal 32 mm Hg blood capillary pressure and may produce irreversible tissue changes when applied constantly for two hours (5). In addi-

139

tion, the shearing forces on the skin of the frail elderly in a sitting position is greater than with younger persons.

The usual location for a pressure sore is the skin over a bony prominence of the lower vertebrae, hips, and heels. Less frequently involved areas are the occiput, earlobes, scapulae, spinous process of the midback and iliac crest.

Pressure sores are classified into four stages (6): Stage 1 – Reddened area that does not disappear when pressure is relieved; Stage 2 – Skin blister or superficial break in the skin; Stage 3 – Skin break with deep tissue involvement and exposure of subcutaneous tissue; Stage 4 – Skin break with deep tissue involvement and exposure of muscle and bone. Sometimes a small erythematous area or a small eschar (thick, black crust) may hide a large deep ulcerated cavity. Removal of the eschar and probing of the cavity may reveal a foul smelling necrotic abscess. The degree of undermining of the skin can be determined with a probe or a cotton swab.

PREVENTION

Prevention of decubitus ulcers is far more effective in time and cost saving for the elderly person in a health care institution than is any treatment regimen once the ulcer develops. Despite general awareness and concern by health care providers, the continuing occurrence of decubitus ulcers reflects the failure to anticipate high risk patients and to institute preventive measures. An assessment scale for screening (Figure 10.1) addresses the major risk factors contributing to the formation of pressure sores (3). From this data, the staff can set priorities for working with the high-risk elderly and direct interventions to the underlying risk factors, e.g., nutrition, incontinence and removal of pressure and friction sources.

Prevention encompasses pressure relief, skin care, mobility, adequate nutrition, patient and family education. The dangers of bed rest are well recognized, so elderly individuals who are not seriously ill should be kept out of bed and active. Unfortunately, the hazard of the sitting position for development of decubiti is not commonly known; it is not unusual for elderly to be sitting for longer intervals without position shifts. Periodic tipping of the wheelchair backwards by 20 degrees can significantly increase blood flow by reducing pressure over bony prominances (7). The

FIGURE 10.1

RISK ASSESSMENT FOR PRESSURE SORES

NAME	DATE	PHYSICAL CONDITION	MENTAL CONDITION	ACTIVITY	MOBILITY	INCONTINENT	TOTAL SCORE
		4–Good 3–Fair 2–Poor 1–Very poor	4–Alert 3–Apathetic 2–Confused 1–Comatose	4–Ambulant 3–Walk/Help 2–Chair-bound 1–Bedfast	4–Full activity 3–Slight limit 2–Needs assist. 1–Immobile	4–None 3–Occasional ($<$ 2X/24 hr) 2–Usual 1–No control	

NOTE: Patients with a total score of $\leq$ 14 should be considered at risk to develop pressure sores and those $<$ 12 are at very high risk. Modified from reference 3.

every-two-hour turning and positioning regimen commonly practiced prevents pressure and tissue ischemia. However, two-hour positioning regimens often are not feasible because of staffing problems and the potentially negative impact on the elderly person of frequent nocturnal awakenings and the pain of gross position changes. Numerous mechanical aids, such as the alternating pressure mattress, "egg carton" mattress, sheepskin, gel pad, and flotation pad, have been developed to aid in these problem areas. However, these devices may have negative consequences if they are used incorrectly by staff. The staff may rely on these aids as a substitute for turning patients and become lax in the vigorous and attentive, ongoing assessment which is required for decubitus prevention and care. The sheekskin or "egg carton" mattress can increase friction forces if the individual is pulled against them rather than lifted. The flotation pad and alternating pressure mattress loses its effectiveness when covered with tightly fitted sheets, thereby increasing skin maceration.

TREATMENT

All treatments for decubitus ulcers include the reduction of pressure, friction, moisture, and shearing forces. This becomes progressively more difficult as the number of decubiti increases and the possible body positions decrease. Mechanical aids become important in augmenting turning, positioning, and padding when the elderly person has more than one decubitus. The prone position is effective in reducing pressure over most of the high-risk areas, but it is used with the frail elderly too infrequently. Staff members generally cite client discomfort or limited tolerance because of impaired respiratory function and joint mobility. Careful attention to padding and adequate staff to assist in quickly and gently accomplishing position change often can rectify the problem.

Treatment is often directed only at the pressure sore with neglect of important mobility and nutritional factors. Activity is beneficial if done with caution to avoid friction, shearing forces, and excessive energy demands on the client. This activity increases peristalsis and appetite, stimulates circulation to affected areas, and maintains or improves mobility required for position changes through general muscle strengthening and joint range of motion. Adequate calories and protein for weight maintenance, or weight gain is recommended for individuals with decubitus ulcers (8). The dietician may suggest changes in the diet to increase caloric intake. In some circumstances a nasogastric tube may be necessary to assure adequate protein and calories. Rest periods, oral care, and pain management intervention prior to meals also are effective strategies for improving food intake. Various vitamins and minerals frequently are used to supplement nutritional deficiencies. Much study is being directed at the role of vitamins, minerals, and trace elements in improving wound healing. Zinc supplements have been associated with an increased rate of wound healing and improved appetite, but results are not consistent. Ascorbic acid supplementation did effectively reduce the healing time of decubitus ulcers among a small group of predominantly elderly patients (9). Studies are not conclusive and must await further confirmation. Correction of anemia and edema hastens healing of pressure sores.

Treatments directed at the decubitus ulcer are numerous. The lack of a systematic, well-controlled study of most treatments makes it impossible to thoroughly evaluate any one for its efficacy. However, there are some standard acceptable practices. A physiological solution of saline and water or Ringer's solution is used to cleanse a wound that is free of necrotic tissue. If the wound is necrotic, hydrogen peroxide or povidone-iodine (Betadine) are useful cleansing agents. These substances must be rinsed with saline and water to avoid damage to tissue. Topical cleansing to remove debris and reduce the risk of infection is used with all stages of decubiti. The use of commercial soaps, alcohol and other astringents such as witch hazel are not advocated as they can cause damage to the epidermis (10). Whirlpool therapy is another popular method for cleansing wounds.

Protective agents form a shield over the skin and frequently are used in the prevention of decubiti and treatment of stage 1 and 2 ulcers. Some examples include: karaya paste, Stomahesive, Op-site, lotions, zinc, and silicone creams. Granulex also is used as a protective agent for stage 1 and 2 ulcers, but in addition it has debriding and bacteriocidal action (11). Dressings reduce client discomfort and wound contamination, but they also create additional skin irritation from the tape, promote skin maceration, and limit early detection of skin deterioration. Op-site, a transparent polyurethane dressing, promotes healing by maintaining a moist environment which accelerates granulation and epithelialization. By preventing eschar formation, epidermal migration is enhanced. Normal body fluids and cells involved in healing are sealed against the ulcer, and bacterial contamination is controlled (12). Karaya paste and Stomahesive function in a similar fashion, although they are not transparent. These protective agents require careful attention to skin preparation and are not recommended for use with ulcers having thick eschar formation or anaerobic bacterial contamination. Silicone creams and hospital lotions have not been shown to be effective in the prevention and treatment of decubitus ulcers (10). In general, ointments, powders, and pastes are usually unsuccessful in facilitating healing of ulcers.

Electrical stimulation, ultraviolet light, and massage are used to stimulate circulation and thereby improve oxygenation to areas of tissue ischemia. All require precautions to avoid traumatizing the area through over-vigorous massage or burns. Ultraviolet light has some bacteriocidal action and also stimulates healing by causing increased blood flow to the involved area. It has been used effectively with a small group of patients in the healing of superficial decubitus ulcers (13).

For healing to occur with stage 2 and 3 ulcers the debris, eschar, and infections must be eliminated. Gelatin sponges and packing of ulcers with various dressings control eschar formation and limit superficial healing prior to granulation of deep tissue. Debrisan, Granulex, Elase, and Cadexomer Iodine are chemical agents which reduce bacteria levels by absorbing and removing exudate and debris. A daily topical application of Cadexomer Iodine, a debriding and antiseptic agent, was found to improve healing significantly and to reduce pain more effectively than standard saline dressings and enzymatic preparations (14). Duoderm, a hydroactive dressing that interacts with exudate to form a soft moist gel that protects the ulcer bed is reported to be effective in promoting healing but has not had extensive trial.

Stage 3 and 4 decubiti are potentially life-threatening for the frail elderly person. Serious disturbances in fluid, electrolyte, and protein-nitrogen balance can occur with a large amount of serum loss. The support measures previously described must be implemented, maintained, and periodically re-evaluated. There is much potential for the development of massive infection and septicemia. Since the skin is not sterile, it is not unusual for cutaneous infections, with purulent drainage and signs of inflammation, to develop. Caregivers must be alert for symptoms which indicate that the client is unable to deal effectively with the infection, such as increased fever, confusion, lethargy, anorexia, purulent drainage, and extension of the decubitus. A wound culture is indicated if antibiotic treatment is to be initiated (15). Osteomyelitis (infection in the bone) may occur beneath a pressure sore and if untreated can become chronic and delay wound healing and recovery (16).

REFERENCES

1. Barbenel, JC; Jordon, MM; Nichol, SM, *et al.*: Incidence of Pressure Sores in the Greater Glasgow Health Board Area. *Lancet, 2:*548, 1977.

2. Reuler, J; Cooney, T: Pressure Sores. In *Geriatric Medicine: Medical, Psychiatric and Pharmacological Topics,* Vol. I, Cassel, C and Walsh, J (Eds.). New York: Springer-Verlag, 1984, pp. 508-516.

3. Norton, D; McLaren, R; Exton-Smith, AN: *An Investigation of Geriatric Nursing Problems in Hospitals.* London: Churchill Livingston, (1962, reissued) 1975, pp. 194-236.

4. Lowthian, P: A Review of Pressure Sore Pathogenesis. *Nurs Times,* 117-121, 1982.

5. Reuler, J. Cooney, T: The Pressure Sore: Pathophysiology and Principles of Management, *Ann Inter Med, 94:*661, 1981.

6. Shea, JD: Pressure Sores: Classification and Management. *Clin Ortho, 112:*89, 1975.

7. Bennett, L: Skin Blood Flow in Seated Geriatric Patients. *Arch Phys Med Rehab, 62:*392, 1981.

8. Natow, A: Nutrition in Prevention and Treatment of Decubitus Ulcers. *Top Clin Nurs,* p. 39, 1983.

9. Taylor, TV, *et al.*: Ascorbic Acid Supplementation in the Treatment of Pressure Sores. *Lancet, 1:*544, 1974.

10. Berecek, K: Treatment of Decubitus Ulcers. *Nurs Clin N Am, 10:*171, 1975.

11. Yucel, VE; Basmajian, JF: Decubitus Ulcers: Healing Effect of an Enzymatic Spray. *Arch Phys Med Rehab, 55:* , 1974.

12. Ahmed, MD: Op-site for Decubitus Care. *Am J Nurs,* 61-64, 1982.

13. Willis, E, *et al.*: A Randomized Placebo-controlled Trial of Ultraviolet Light in the Treatment of Superficial Pressure Sores. *J Am Geriat Soc, 31:* 131, 1983.

14. Moberg, S, *et al.*: A Randomized Trial of Codexomer Iodine in Decubitus Ulcers, *J Am Geriat Soc, 31:*462, 1983.

15. Gurevich, I: Infected Decubiti: The Problem of Patient Placement and Care. *Top Clin Nurs,* 55-63, 1983 (July).

16. Sugarman, B; Hawls, S; Musher, DM, *et al.*: Osteomyelitis Beneath Pressure Sores. *Arch Intern Med, 143:*683, 1983.

CHAPTER 11

OSTEOPOROSIS

BRITTLE BONES

Osteoporosis is characterized by a decrease in the total amount of bone. Bone tissue that remains is normally mineralized but the thickness and number of bone trabeculae has decreased. Therefore, osteoporotic bone is similar to normal bone except that there is less of it. A consequence of osteoporosis is increased bony fragility and predisposition to fractures even with minimal or no trauma. Fractures are responsible for 5% of hospitalized patients over age 65 in the United States, and this increases to 10.2% after age 85. Nearly 4% of the population 85 years or over sustain a serious fracture each year (1). About 1 million fractures occur annually in American women over age 45. Approximately 70% of these are related to osteoporosis. The three major sites of fracture involve the spinal vertebra, hip and wrist. The costs in terms of functional disability and financial outlay are enormous.

Cortical bone surrounds an inner porous trabecular bone. With aging there is a decline in cortical bone mass and trabecular bone volume. In an aging person, sex steroid deficiency, decrease in calcium intake and a decline in physical activity may be responsible so that it is difficult to determine the effects due to aging alone on bone (2). Some believe that loss of bone mass should not be attributed to aging per se but that it is entirely the effects of a decline in sex steroids.

Bone is continuously remodeled through the process of breakdown (resorption) and formation. When breakdown exceeds formation, bone becomes thinner and osteoporosis results. A decline in bone mass begins in both sexes at about the age of 30 to 35. However, men have a larger bone mass early in life than women and it declines more slowly with age so that symptomatic osteoporosis seldom develops until advanced old age. Decreases in bone mass in men are delayed until age 60 years, after which the rate of bone loss is 0.3 to 0.5% per year.

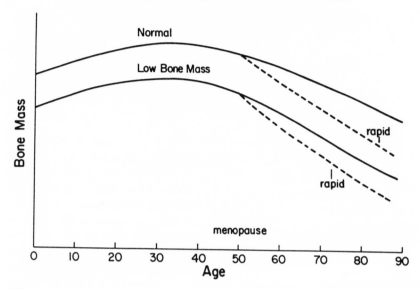

Figure 11.1. Women have lower bone density than men. Loss of bone begins about age 30 to 35 years in both sexes. In addition to loss of bone with aging, loss of ovarian function accelerates bone loss in some women. Removal of ovaries (surgical menopause) prior to biological menopause hastens onset of osteoporosis. Thin women have smaller bones than obese women and are more vulnerable to fractures. Black women have larger bones, therefore are less subject to fractures.

Osteoporosis most often occurs in post-menopausal women (Figure 11.1). Women lose bone most rapidly in the first five to six years following menopause. The rate of bone loss decreases after age 65 and becomes similar to that of men. The rate of total bone loss is approximately 0.5% per year after the age of 40; however, in postmenopausal women the rate accelerates to 1% or more per year for about ten years (3). It decreases to 0.5% per year thereafter.

In the United States, dietary deficiency of calcium is a major cause of osteoporosis and may be responsible for bone loss that begins after age 30 in normal women. Other important risk factors are shown in Table 11.1.

TABLE 11.1
MAJOR RISK FACTORS IN OSTEOPOROSIS

1. Sex steroids
   Women
       Menopause
       Oophorectomy
   Men
       Androgen deficiency
2. Aging
3. Immobilization
4. Smoking
5. Thin women
6. Nutritional deficiency
   Calcium/phosphorus
7. High protein diet
8. Drugs
   Corticosteroids
   Heparin (⟩ 6 months)
   Aluminum–containing antacids

IMMOBILIZATION

After several weeks of immobilization, significant bone loss occurs due to lack of weight bearing activity. A bedfast patient has increased urinary loss of calcium and decreased absorption of calcium from the diet. Removing the stress of gravity from the skeleton with bedrest accelerates a breakdown (resorption) of bone and produces osteoporosis or worsens an existing osteoporosis. On the other hand, exercise significantly improves calcium retention in post–menopausal women (4). Weight bearing exercise such as walking or jogging and an adequate dietary intake of calcium slows the rate of bone loss and may somewhat increase bone mass. However, once bone has been lost it is virtually impossible to build it back to normal in aging people. Therefore, prevention of loss must be vigorously endorsed.

SMOKING

An increased incidence of osteoporosis is found in cigarette smokers. The mechanism is unknown. Thin white women of Northern European extraction especially if they have a low dietary calcium intake and are smokers are at high risk for osteoporosis.

ALUMINUM-CONTAINING ANTACIDS

Aluminum-containing antacids may lead to loss of calcium and phosphorus and increases breakdown (resorption) of bone (6). Aluminum combines with phosphorus in the intestine causing increased fecal phosphorus excretion. The resultant decrease in intestinal phosphorus absorption subsequently results in a decrease in serum phosphorus and a low phosphorus excretion in the urine. Bone resorption is induced to release phosphorus from bone to replace the low levels in the serum and body fluids. The loss of phosphorus from bone is accompanied by calcium which is then excreted in urine. A high dietary intake of calcium and phosphorus during the use of aluminum-containing antacids can prevent bone loss.

CLINICAL FEATURES

The first clinical manifestation of reduced bone mass is usually a fracture of the wrist or hip or a vertebral crush fracture. The vertebrae are primarily composed of the mesh-like trabecular bone and after years of bone loss the vertebrae become more porous and weak and in time may actually collapse (Figure 11.2). Vertebral fractures may occur spontaneously, the weakened bones collapsing under the weight of the body. More commonly, however, they occur with ordinary activity such as lifting a chair, heavy box, a child or opening a window. With the collapse of several vertebrae, dorsal kyphosis occurs producing a loss of height. A recent vertebral fracture causes severe localized back pain which may radiate anteriorly into the chest or abdomen. It is usually relieved by lying down and it improves over a period of one to two months. Neurological signs are rare.

Hip fractures are extremely common especially in women (7). Often, the injury is caused by slipping on a throw rug, tripping over a stair or falling in a bathtub. However, a hip fracture may occur with no apparent cause, the fracture itself causing the fall. The consequences of a hip fracture are serious. The incidence of fractures approximately doubles every five years after the age of 45. Less than 50% of hip fracture patients recover normal function and about 30% of hip fractures in women over age 65 will result directly in premature death.

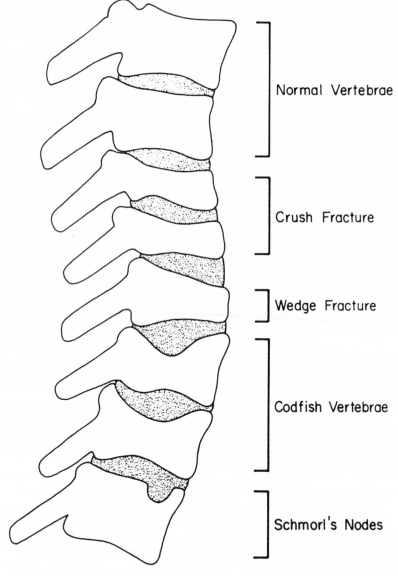

Figure 11.2. Compression and compaction of thoracic or lumbar vertebrae initially produces biconcave vertebrae with ballooning of the intervertebral disc hence are called codfish vertebrae. The nucleus pulposis may herniate into the vertebral body (Schmorl's node). Anterior compression of the vertebral body produces a wedge fracture. Total collapse of the vertebral body is called a crushed fracture.

PREVENTION AND MANAGEMENT

In women over age 30, preventive measures include weight bearing exercises such as walking or jogging, and cessation of smoking, drinking alcohol, coffee and cola drinks. Women over age 30 should ingest about 1 gram of elemental calcium per day in their diet which can be accomplished by drinking 1 quart of skim milk or taking calcium in the form of calcium carbonate (40% elemental calcium). Calcium supplements are effective in retarding age–related bone loss (8) and may also decrease the fracture rate in osteoporosis (9). A total calcium intake of approximately 1000 mg/day is considered adequate in younger women to forestall bone loss. Women, apprehensive about gaining weight by consuming dairy products must supplement their approximatley 500 mg daily intake with calcium tablets to achieve adequate intake. Older people need even a higher intake because of absorption of calcium decreases with age. The post–menopausal woman who is not taking estrogens requires about 1500 mg/day. If estrogens are administered a calcium intake of 1000 mg/day is sufficient. A glass of milk contains about 200 mg of calcium. Cheese, sardines, nuts, and leafy vegetables are good sources of calcium. Some older people with osteoporosis have lactase deficiency (lactose intolerance) and develop diarrhea, abdominal cramps and bloating from intestinal gas because they are unable to split the sugar, lactose, found in milk, ice cream and other dairy products. The use of calcium supplement (tablets) circumvents this problem.

Calcium carbonate tablets containing 250 to 500 mg of elemental calcium are the cheapest calcium supplements available. Tums contain 500 mg calcium carbonate per tablet (40% elemental calcium) and, therefore, about five tablets are equivalent to one gram of elemental calcium per day. Other forms of calcium have less elemental calcium and require ingesting a greater number of tablets to achieve comparable results. Calcium gluconate and calcium lactate tablets contain 90 and 104 mg of elemental calcium respectively. Vitamin D in low doses (400 international units per day) is safe and helpful for women with poor dietary intake. This may be supplied in a combined preparation with calcium or in a multivitamin tablet.

Oral estrogen therapy prevents loss of bone mass in osteoporosis and most importantly decreases the number of fractures (8, 10). If started early enough after menopause, estrogens have, in fact, increased bone mass in some individuals. The dose of conjugated estrogen necessary to preserve bone mass is 0.625 mg per day. To be most effective, estrogen therapy should be started as soon as possible after the beginning of menopause, preferably within the first three years and continued for approximately ten years. The benefit of prevention of fractures must be weighed against the risks of estrogen therapy such as endometrial carcinoma and gall bladder disease (11). Estrogen administration stimulates the endometrium and is associated with an increased incidence of endometrial carcinoma. This risk may be reduced by appropriate attention to vaginal bleeding, periodic pelvic examination with vaginal smears and recently Medroxyprogesterone intermittently to reduce endometrial hyperplasia and consequently the risk of carcinoma (12). Presently, estrogen therapy cannot be recommended for all post–menopausal women but should be considered for those women who have high risk of developing severe osteoporosis and fractures. This includes women who have had their ovaries removed surgically, those who have early menopause and especially slender, white women who have been cigarette smokers and likely have osteopenia. The incidence of cholelithiasis is doubled in women taking estrogen therapy. Some patients are unwilling to accept the discomfort of breast swelling, renewal of vaginal bleeding or the risk of endometrial cancer or gall bladder disease with estrogen therapy.

Anabolic androgens such as stanozolol slows the rate of bone loss and has been purported to restore previously lost bone mass in patients with post–menopausal osteoporosis (13). It is usually administered daily in cycles of three weeks followed by one week drug-free period. Androgen steroid therapy is combined with a calcium intake of at least 1000 mg daily. Liver abnormalities may cause elevation of the serum alkaline phosphatase and bilirubin levels. Some women may find steroids unpleasant because of growth of facial and body hair, acne, ankle edema and husky voice.

Sodium fluoride has been used in conjunction with an increased calcium intake, vitamin D and estrogens to increase bone mass. However, adverse effects such as arthritis, vomiting and anemia limit its use.

REFERENCES

1. Wylie, CM: Hospitalization for Fractures and Bone Loss in Adults. *Pub Hlth Rep, 92:*33, 1977.

2. Heaney, RP; Gallagher, JC; Johnston, CC; Neer R, *et al.*: Calcium Nutrition and Bone Health in the Elderly. *Am J Clin Nutr, 36:*986-1003, 1982.

3. Smith, DM; Khairi, MRA; Norton, J, *et al.*: Age and Activity Effects on Rate of Bone Mineral Loss. *J Clin Invest, 58:*716, 1976.

4. Aloia, JF; Cohn, SH; Ostuni, JA, *et al.*: Prevention of Involutional Bone Loss by Exercise. *Ann Intern Med, 89:*356, 1978.

5. Daniell, HW: Osteoporosis of the Slender Smoker; Vertebral Compression Fractures and Loss of Metacarpal Cortex in Relation to Postmenopausal Cigarette Smoking and Lack of Obesity. *Arch Intern Med, 136:*298, 1976.

6. Spencer, H; Kramer, L: Antacid-induced Calcium Loss. *Arch Intern Med, 143:*657, 1983.

7. Wallace, WA: The Increasing Incidence of Fractures of the Proximal Femur: An Orthopaedic Epidemic. *Lancet, 1:*1413, 1983.

8. Recker, RR; Saville, PD; Heaney, RP: Effect of Estrogens and Calcium Carbonate on Bone Loss in Postmenopausal Women. *Ann Int Med, 87:*649, 1977.

9. Riggs, BL; Seeman, E; Hodgson, SF, *et al.*: Effect of the Fluoride/Calcium Regimen on Vertebral Fracture Occurrence in Postmenopausal Osteoporosis: Comparison with Conventional Therapy. *N Eng J Med, 306:*446, 1982.

10. Weiss, NS; Ure, CL; Ballard, JH; Williams, AR, *et al.*: Decreased Risk of Fracture of the Hip and Lower Forearm with Postmenopausal Use of Estrogen. *N Eng J Med, 303:*1195, 1980.

11. Weinstein, MC: Estrogen Use in Postmenopausal Women: Costs, Risks and Benefits. *N Eng J Med, 303:*308-316, 1980.

12. Whitehead, MJ; Townsend, PT; Pryse-Davis, J, *et al.*: Effects of Estrogens and Progestins on the Biochemistry and Morphology of the Postmenopausal Endometrium. *N Eng J Med, 304:*1599, 1981.

13. Krane, S: Disorders of Bone Formation and Resorption. In *Scientific American Medicine*, Rubenstein, E. (Ed.). New York, 1983.

CHAPTER 12

THE EFFECT OF HEAT
AND COLD IN THE OLD

In old people, autonomic nervous system function is reduced. One sequelae is impairment of thermoregulation (the body's "thermostat" is less efficient) which makes the older person more susceptible to hypothermia during prolonged exposure to a cold environment and conversely, heat stroke or heat exhaustion during prolonged exposure to a warm environment. The regulation of body temperature, therefore, is more unstable in the elderly and the body is less able to respond to heat or cold.

HYPOTHERMIA

On exposure to a cold environment, the body normally protects itself by conserving heat through constriction of blood vessels of the skin and by shivering which increases muscular activity. Older people don't shiver as effectively to generate body heat because they have less muscle mass. Additionally, the frail elderly have lost much of the protective layer of fat under the skin that helps keep people warm. Frail older people are sometimes not aware that they are becoming cold (1). Prolonged exposure to cold is particularly harmful to the elderly who are more likely to have autonomic dysfunction. Autonomic dysfunction is found in approximately 10% of "normal" old people. The combination of orthostatic hypotension, abnormalities in vasoconstriction and low body temperature suggests that an autonomic neuropathy may predispose some older people to hypothermia in cool environments that are tolerated by others (2, 3). Even mild decreases in room temperature below 65°F (18.3°C) can cause significant reduction in core body temperature to be hazardous. Factors that predispose to hypothermia are shown in Table 12.1. Hypothermia (an internal body temperature below 95°F (35°C) is likely to

```
                    TABLE 12.1
         RISK FACTORS FOR HYPOTHERMIA

  • Environmental factors
        Freezing weather
        Wet clothing, wind
        Inadequate heating in home
  • Low income, living alone, frailty
  • Insufficient clothing
  • Disorders that cause immobility or falls
        Stroke
        Arthritis
        Parkinson's Disease
  • Drugs
        Alcohol
        Phenothiazines
        Barbiturates
        Antidepressants
  • Hypothyroidism
```

develop in an older person living alone especially if unable to afford adequate heating, or who after falling is unable to get up. Other persons at risk are those who use drugs such as barbiturates, phenothiazines, antidepressants or during general anesthesia. A demented individual who wanders in freezing weather or an alcoholic who may sleep under a bridge or by the side of the road may develop hypothermia. Hypothyroidism is also commonly associated with hypothermia (4).

Clinical Features

The patient usually is pale. There may be swelling of the face, slow cerebration, a husky voice and sluggish reflexes, a constellation of findings simulating hypothyroidism. The abdominal wall is cold to the touch. Confusion and disorientation occurs when the body temperature is below 90°F (32°C). The pulse rate falls to 40–50 beats/min, and there is a decrease in blood pressure. Initially, on exposure to cold, shivering and diuresis occurs but as the body temperature drops to 32°C, shivering ceases and muscular rigidity occurs. Slow, shallow breathing ensues.

Hypothermia may be missed using standard thermometers but is detected by taking the rectal temperature with a low reading thermometer or by measuring the temperature of freshly voided urine (4, 5, 6).

Protective Measures

Hypothermia usually affects persons living alone and is often associated with immobility and falls. Therefore, maintaining the room temperature at 65°F (18.3°C) may alleviate part of the problem. Dressing with warm clothing including sweaters and perhaps emulating old-timers who wore nightcaps (since it has been shown that significant heat loss occurs from an uncovered head) and avoidance of drugs that predispose to hypothermia are effective preventive measures.

Management

General supportive measures such as warmed intravenous fluid and electrolytes, correction of metabolic acidosis, and hypoxia, monitoring for cardiac dysrhythmias and the use of rewarming techniques are effective (6). Rewarming should not be done rapidly. Table 12.2 shows some rewarming measures.

TABLE 12.2
TREATMENT MEASURES

- Remove from windy area
- Replace wet clothing
- Wrap with warm blanket
- Use hot water bottle wrapped in towel or electric heating pads
- Warm fluids orally, if alert
- Specific rewarming techniques
    Intragastric or colonic irrigation
    Peritoneal dialysis
    Extracorporeal blood rewarming
    Inhalation rewarming

HEAT STROKE

Hypothermia in the elderly, the old in the cold, has received considerable publicity. The effects of heat, on the other hand, is devastating and more common. Hot weather can cause serious illness in elderly people called heat stroke. The elderly population is at greater risk to develop heat stroke and mortality increases with advancing age during heat waves (7, 8, 9). Marked and especially sudden increases in core body temperature can result in tissue

TABLE 12.3
RISK FACTORS FOR HEAT STROKE

- Alcoholism
- Drugs
    Anticholinergics
    Phenothiazines
    Antidepressants
- Living in top story, poor ventilation
- Crowded rooms in older nursing homes
- Dehydration
- Infection with fever

damage. Epidemics of heat stroke in several cities have killed hundreds and has increased deaths in elderly people suffering from underlying diseases, a condition known as heat aggravated disease (9). Debilitating diseases predisposing to heat stroke are congestive heart failure, dementia, diabetes, neurological disorders, and chronic obstructive pulmonary disease. Table 12.3 shows factors associated with heat stroke (10). Older people should be given specific instructions to prevent heat stroke in warm climates (Table 12.4).

The onset of symptoms is usually sudden, often a patient who has been well before retiring for the night is found with delirium, and rapid progression to coma. Seizures may occur. Average rectal temperature is 41.3°C. Some may sweat but most do not. A rapid pulse rate is almost always present. Hyperventila-

TABLE 12.4
PROTECTIVE MEASURES IN HOT WEATHER

- Drink lots of water — 6-8 glasses per day
- Wear lightweight and light-colored clothing
- Rest frequently in a shady or cool place (basement, air conditioned room)
- Avoid exertion or exercise especially in the afternoon
- Avoid prolonged exposure to sunlight
- If you live alone, be in daily contact with friends, relatives or neighbors — even by telephone
- If you develop weakness, nausea, vomiting, headache, dizziness, shortness of breath and a feeling of warmth, contact your doctor

tion causes respiratory alkalosis, Dehydration is frequently present and hypokalemia is common. Increase in blood lactate occurs which causes metabolic acidosis. Acute renal failure may occur in severe cases. Liver function tests increase, reflecting damage to liver cells. Muscle damage occurs in those who have exerted themselves.

Treatment consists of moving patients to a cool environment, and cooling the body with ice or cold water, intravenous fluids to correct water and electrolyte deficits, management of shock, prevention of aspiration, and treating renal failure.

Heat exhaustion is a mild form of hyperpyrexia causing lightheadedness or syncope due to low blood volume. It is a warning of impending heat stroke.

REFERENCES

1. Fox, RH; MacGibbon, R; Davies, L, et al.: Problems of the old and the cold. Br Med J, 1:21, 1973.
2. Collins, KJ; Dore, C; Exton-Smith, AN, et al.: Accidental hypothermia and impaired temperature homeostasis in the elderly. Br Med J, 1:353, 1977.
3. Exton-Smith, AN: Disturbances of autonomic regulation. In Recent Advances in Geriatrics, Isaacs, B (Ed.). New York: Churchill Livingstone, 1978, pp. 85-100.
4. Reuler, JB: Hypothermia: Pathophysiology, clinical setting and management. Ann Intern Med, 89:519, 1978.
5. Fox, RH; Woodward, PM; Fry, AJ, et al.: Diagnosis of accidental hypothermia of the elderly. Lancet, 1:424, 1971.
6. Reuler, J: Hypothermia, In Geriatric Medicine: Medical, Psychiatric and Pharmacological Topics, Vol. I, Cassel, C and Walsh, J (Eds.). New York: Springer-Verlag, 1984, pp. 486-492.
7. Applegate, WB; Runyan, JW; Brasfield, L, et al.: Analysis of the 1980 heat wave in Memphis. J Am Geriatr Soc, 29:337, 1981.
8. Hart, GR; Anderson, RJ; Crumpler, CP, et al.: Epidemic classical heat stroke: Clinical characteristics and course of 28 patients. Medicine, 61:189, 1982.
9. Jones, TS; Liang, AP; Kilbourne, EM, et al.: Morbidity and mortality associated with the July 1980 heat wave in St. Louis and Kansas City, MO. JAMA, 247:3327, 1982.
10. Kilbourne, EM; Choi, K; Jones, TS, et al.: Risk factors for heat stroke. A case-control study. JAMA, 247:3332, 1982.

Part 3
STRATEGIES IN MANAGEMENT

CHAPTER 13

CEREBROVASCULAR PROBLEMS

TRANSIENT ISCHEMIC ATTACKS

Transient ischemic attacks (TIAs, "little strokes") are due to decreased blood flow to parts of the brain comparable to angina pectoris (chest pain) produced by diminished blood flow through coronary arteries to heart muscle. They are most common in the elderly with a peak incidence in the seventh decade. TIAs serve as a forewarning of impending stroke. If untreated, about one third will suffer a completed stroke, one third will continue to have TIAs and one third will recover without getting a stroke (1). Treatment of TIAs can prevent stroke but unfortunately many people do not see a physician until they have developed a stroke.

A TIA is a sudden episode of neurologic dysfunction usually lasting 2 to 5 minutes but never more than 24 hours and subsides completely. TIAs result from blood clots on atheromatous placques in the major vessels of the neck which interfere with blood supply to the brain. Small parts of the clot break off (microemboli) and lodge in a small artery of the brain to cause symptoms. TIAs are classified according to their source, that is, carotid artery or vertebral artery insufficiency. Any emboli from either of these vessels will reach areas of the brain supplied by the particular vessel involved. Therefore, symptoms are different depending on which vessel is involved. Prognosis and treatment also differ.

TABLE 13.1
KINDS OF STROKE

Ischemic stroke
    Thrombus in a cerebral artery
    Embolus in a cerebral artery

Cerebral hemorrhage
    Bleeding in brain tissue
    Bleeding in the subarachnoid space

Carotid Artery Syndrome

Symptoms are typically any one or combination of the following:

1. *Total or partial loss of vision in one eye (amaurosis fugax)* — the patient describes a sudden loss of vision as if a shade is pulled down over the eye, the episode lasting from seconds to minutes. Vision in the opposite eye is unchanged. Fundoscopic examination may reveal refractile orange–yellow cholesterol emboli or a whitish–gray embolus in the retinal arteriole blocking the blood flow.
2. *Aphasia.* The patient can think of some words but is unable to say certain words and may not understand what is being said to him.
3. *Motor disturbance.* Weakness, paralysis or clumsiness of arm, leg, or face on one side.
4. *Sensory defects.* Numbness or altered sensations such as tingling, burning, pins and needles in limbs and on one side of the face.
5. *Homonymous hemianopia.* Loss of one half of the corresponding visual field in both eyes (upper or lower half, right or left).

On physical examination, the carotid pulsation on the involved side may be reduced. A bruit over the carotid artery suggests arterial stenosis. However, the absence of a bruit does not rule out carotid artery stenosis.

Vertebrobasilar Artery Syndrome

Symptoms stem from involvement of the posterior portion of the brain, the occipital lobes and brainstem and are, therefore, sometimes bilateral.

1. *Bilateral visual disturbance* described as dim, gray or blurred vision or total blindness. It may be described as a shade pulled down over both eyes. Diplopia (double vision) may occur.
2. *Slurring dysarthria.* Difficulty in which the speech is slurred or distorted like that of an alcoholic drunk, difficulty swallowing, numbness around mouth, weakness, loss of sensation and paresthesias of all four limbs are symptoms of brainstem involvement.
3. *Drop attacks.* Patient suddenly loses muscle tone in the legs and abruptly falls without losing consciousness.

Patients with vertebrobasilar TIAs may develop attacks in relation to posture, or body movements such as hyperextension of the head which may cause further mechanical obstruction of the artery.

Management of TIAs

The occurrence of any transient episodes suggesting TIA should be considered a warning of impending stroke. Medical treatment with either aspirin or warfarin is indicated for patients with normal arteriograms, multiple vascular lesions and vertebrobasilar lesions because of extent of involvement. Some physicians use anticoagulants such as warfarin for an initial TIA in the first two months. In the latter situation, or when aspirin fails, they are usually used for two to three months although some experts recommend long-term therapy (1, 2). However, warfarin can be a dangerous drug in an elderly patient and, therefore, should be used only in select cases. Aspirin used as an antiplatelet agent for TIAs is the drug of choice (1, 3). Aspirin is the most common drug in the treatment of TIA.

Surgical treatment (endarterectomy) by removing atheromatous plaques and blood clots from inside the artery is effective for patients with significant carotid artery stenosis (usually greater than 80%). Angiography followed by endarterectomy is indicated for patients who are good medical risks. The operation apparently reduces the frequency of transient ischemic attacks and may decrease the development of future cerebral infarction (3).

STROKE

Last year approximately 750,000 new cases of stroke occurred in the United States (1). Nearly one third die (approximately 250,000) annually from stroke. It ranks only behind heart disease and cancer as a cause of death among Americans. Even more alarming is the residual disability, 16% of survivors will spend the rest of their lives in institutions, another 20% will need assistance to ambulate, and 31% will need assistance with self-care (4). There are about 2.5 million disabled stroke survivors in this country. Strokes incapacitate far more people than they kill and are, therefore, responsible for long-term functional disability in considerable numbers of people.

Major risk factors for stroke are the same as those for athero-sclerosis. The most important established risk factor is high blood pressure. Another potentially treatable risk factor is heart disease especially embolic cerebrovascular lesions from heart wall or valvular thrombi which are more likely in atrial fibrillation, myo-cardial infarction and valvular heart disease. Other important risk factors are age, diabetes mellitis, and cigarette smoking. Con-trolling high blood pressure, cessation of smoking and reducing risk factors are preventive measures employed to lower the inci-dence of stroke.

There is evidence that the incidence of stroke has been drop-ping during the past 30 years particularly in the elderly, probably because hypertension, its major cause, is being better treated and possibly because of a decline in salt intake and other dietary measures (5, 6). Not only has the incidence of stroke been declin-ing but there has been a progressive improvement in long-term survival perhaps due to better management of associated condi-tions such as heart disease, treatment of respiratory infection and improvement in functional skills through greater use of rehabili-tation therapy (7). The peak incidence of strokes is in the sixth decade and only about 20% occur before the age of sixty-five.

Interference with the blood supply of the brain causes stroke. Blockage of one of the arteries of the brain or neck by a blood clot (thrombus) or by an embolus (a wandering blood clot) causes poor blood supply (ischemia) in the brain. Cerebral hemorrhage is due to rupture of a blood vessel in the brain of an individual with high blood pressure. By far the most common cause of stroke is cerebral thrombosis or clot formation in a cerebral artery. Nearly half of patients with stroke have had premonitory symptoms of TIA which should be considered a warning sign of a stroke.

A stroke producing a lesion of one side of the brain will result in hemiplegia on the opposite side of the body. Stroke, however, produces more than just hemiplegia. The victim of a stroke will have significant difficulties that impair balance and coordination, sensory perception, memory, cognition and behavior (8, 9). Other accompanying clinical findings usually distinguish dysfunction of the dominant (left) and the nondominant (right) cerebral hemispheres. Speech functions in both right and left-handed people are most often localized in the left cerebral hemi-sphere and a lesion here results in the loss of ability to speak or understand speech (aphasia or dysphasia). On the other hand, a stroke producing a lesion on the right side of the brain causes a

TABLE 13.2
MAJOR DIFFERENCE
BETWEEN RIGHT AND LEFT HEMIPLEGIA

LESION RIGHT BRAIN	LESION LEFT BRAIN
Left hemiplegia	Right hemiplegia
Decreased perception Poor position sense Spatial disorientation Unilateral neglect Impaired judgment Short attention span	Speech and language disorder Aphasia

left hemiplegia. Other accompanying dysfunctions are loss of position sense (proprioception), inability to judge depth and vertical/horizontal orientation in the environment (10). In addition, there is a lack of awareness of the left side of the body unexplained by sensory or visual defects (8, 9). Therefore, with left hemiplegia health professionals must look for functional disabilities which influence rehabilitation efforts. Unilateral neglect may be extreme so that the patient is unaware of people approaching on that side or fails to shave or dress on that side. The patient may deny loss of function and may not recognize their left arm as being their own.

Aphasia is inability to speak or understand the spoken word. It is a sign of a left cerebral lesion and is, therefore, typically associated with right hemiplegia. On the other hand, the patient with left hemiplegia usually has intact language ability. Aphasia may be seen clinically as difficulty to comprehend spoken or written words (receptive or sensory aphasia) or difficulty expressing oneself in speech or writing (expressive aphasia). Often a mixed picture is seen. Reading inability (alexia) and incapability of writing usually accompany aphasia.

Recently, aphasias have been classified as fluent or non–fluent instead of expressive or receptive aphasias. Non–fluent aphasia formerly called expressive or motor aphasia is characterized by slow speech with pauses and hesitation, often with short incomplete phrases. There is inability to name common objects or repeat simple phrases. However, the patient may be able to follow simple commands indicating that some ability to comprehend is intact. On the other hand, fluent aphasia, previously called receptive or sensory aphasia is characterized by incorrect word usage, reversed syllables or even unintelligible speech. Words may be substituted for others, as clock for watch, soap for sink.

Aphasias may be transient and over half of those afflicted recover completely within the first few weeks. The greatest degree of recovery in the remaining aphasics occurs during the first year. Speech therapy and the use of communication aids should be started early.

Dysarthria is a speech disorder in which the patient has an articulation disorder with difficulty speaking clearly and understandably but has no trouble using appropriate words, reading, writing or comprehending what others say.

Visual field defect, homonymous hemianopsia refers to loss of vision of the medial half of one eye and the lateral half of the other. The visual field deficit is on the same side as the hemiplegia. A patient with left hemiplegia and left homonymous hemianopsia has blindness in the corresponding left visual field. Health care providers sometimes forget that the patient ignores activity on the blind side (11). The patient should be positioned in bed so that the uninvolved side views the doorway to the room to help the patient identify visitors. If the patient only eats food from half of the plate he/she may ignore the other half because of the visual defect. The patient must be taught to turn the head to compensate for the defect or to turn the plate during mealtime.

Unilateral visual field neglect develops with damage to the occipital cortex which interprets an object in the opposite visual field. Therefore, an object in the left visual field does not exist with a right–sided occipital lesion and vice versa. Food on one side of the plate is eaten, time is read on one side of a clock.

Apraxia is the inability to execute purposeful movement which cannot be explained by weakness, paralysis, sensory loss, poor comprehension or inattention to commands (12). It is essentially a defect in integrative steps that convert intellectual or sensory stimuli into voluntary movement. With apraxia the patient often cannot plan an integrated motor act such as putting on a sweater. They have difficulty following commands that require an action such as picking up a book, blowing out a match, sticking the tongue out, buttoning a shirt, using a toothbrush or using a comb. The patient can do some of these tasks automatically but has problems when asked specifically to do them. There may be trouble in following instructions from a therapist or a nurse when asked to do a task or imitate a purposeful movement. Patients with apraxia are sometimes suspected of malingering or being uncooperative because they have good strength and have no language impairment. Apraxia makes training such as gait training very difficult.

The patient must be able to comprehend verbal commands in order to perform a movement. The region for comprehension is in the left brain, called Wernicke's area. A command to perform a movement goes to Wernicke's area in the left hemisphere and is transmitted to the left or right side of the brain for control of movement of the appropriate limb. A lesion of the left cerebral hemisphere causes apraxia of the right hand. A lesion of the corpus callosum which connects the right and left cerebral hemispheres and which transmits the message from Wernicke's area of the left brain to the right brain, is responsible for apraxia of the left hand (12). Apraxia is most often bilateral and, therefore, mainly due to a frontal lobe lesion with involvement of the corpus callosum.

Neglect is a disorder of spatial orientation caused by a damaged right parietal lobe. It is a lateralized loss of awareness of the patient's left side and the environment on that side. It, therefore, is associated with left hemiplegia and seldom is seen with right hemiplegia. Because of a lesion in the right parietal lobe, sensory information from the left side of the body is not processed. These patients have considerable difficulty in spatial orientation and are unable to localize stimuli or objects in space. The patient may ignore the left side of the body or environment. It can occur in patients who have no visual field defect. The patient may fail to dress or shave the left side and may be unaware of people approaching on the neglected side. Some patients deny that the left leg or arm is paralyzed. The patient is unaware of the existence of these deficits and, therefore, will not complain about them.

Constructional apraxia describes difficulty with the interpretation of visual clues and their spatial organization such as the inability to draw or construct geometric shapes, drawing, block designs, etc. The task requries more than just skilled hand movements. It also involves integration of spatial relationships. Drawing common geometric designs to test this type of apraxia is often included in the mental status examination (12). Constructional impairment may be associated with diffuse cerebral lesions but most often results from a lesion in the parietal lobe. The right parietal lobe has the highest incidence and the greater severity of defect.

Loss of Position Sense (Proprioception)
and Spatial Relationships

Loss of proprioception and poor spatial perception have a significant effect on rehabilitation of the stroke patient (11). The left hemiplegic patient often has trouble in judging depth and in adjusting to horizontal and vertical cues in the environment. Proprioception or position sensation from muscles, tendons, ligaments and joints courses through posterior columns of the spinal cord to the parietal lobes. Patients with profound proprioceptive loss have considerable difficulty in achieving self-care and usually require longer periods of time for rehabilitation. Usually if recovery does occur it does so within two months after the stroke (10).

Stroke patients may be unable to concentrate for more than a few minutes and may be easily distracted. Weakness and fatigue worsen the ability to concentrate and may interfere with rehabilitative measures. Shorter and more frequent periods of activity are better tolerated and less frustrating for the therapist, nurse or spouse helping with the activity. With recovery the attention span increases. In addition to inability to concentrate, judgment may be impaired and there may be personality changes. The stroke victim is sometimes irritable because of loss of functional capabilities and displays of anger should not be countered with abruptness, scolding or patronizing attitudes.

Apathy or disinterest in participating in any activity may be a barrier to successful rehabilitation. It may be a greater problem with left hemiplegia as is denial of the illness. The patient may refuse assistance or poor motivation may make rehabilitation ineffective. Health professionals should not misinterpret these responses as uncooperativeness of the patient.

Urinary incontinence following a stroke is due to an uninhibited bladder which often improves in time. In addition, immobility or apathy may lead to incontinence. Continence returns in about 50% of incontinent patients in the first six months and a further 18% during the second six months.

The goal of rehabilitation of stroke patients is to make them as self-sufficient as possible. The staff should train patients in self-care. The patient should participate in his/her own care from the beginning. On the other hand, we should recognize our limitations and not waste time and energy on unobtainable goals. If it becomes obvious that the patient will not walk, emphasis should be shifted to the use of a wheelchair and teaching transfer procedures. It is often easier for the staff to perform an activity for the patient such as dressing since allowing the patient to dress may be time consuming. This may encourage an attitude of helplessness, a behavioral pattern that must not be reinforced. At time of discharge family members must be informed about what the patient can do himself and how to assist in self-care. Patients should be encouraged to do as much as possible for themselves and health providers or family should never criticize failure.

Neurological recovery from infirmities of stroke generally takes three to four months and may even continue for six months (11). Slight recovery is sometimes prolonged to one year. Age influences fatality rate for atherosclerotic infarction being three times greater after age 70 in men. Death in the first 30 days after stroke is due to the stroke itself. In long-term survivors cardiovascular disease is the leading cause of death. Cardiovascular disease and hypertension favor stroke recurrence, especially in men (14). Therefore, early treatment of congestive heart failure and elevated blood pressure may influence survival. Treatment of hypertension clearly prevents the initial stroke and is an important aspect of preventing recurrent stroke.

Stroke rehabilitation focuses on prevention of functional disability and restoring the patient to as high a level of independent functioning in his or her environment as possible (15). There is no better example of interdisciplinary team collaboration than with stroke patients. Preventive rehabilitation concentrates on early mobilization as a means to slow muscle atrophy, and loss of strength, reduce spasticity, and to prevent contractures and complications of prolonged bed rest (15). It should start as soon as the patient's conditions is stable. It includes correct positioning and posturing of the patient when in bed or sitting in a chair. This is a 24-hour responsibility to avoid poor hemiplegic posture and loss of mobility (7). It is not sufficient to practice rehabilitation intermittently only in the rehabilitation unit. Activity of daily-living training helps develop skills for self-sufficiency and independent living.

Swallowing difficulties may lead to aspiration. The mouth should be checked for retained food which often accumulates on the affected side. Some patients have difficulty swallowing liquids or flaky foods but are able to swallow foods with firmer consistency. Giving fluid in the form of popsicles provides a bolus that is easier swallowed. Positioning the patient in a sitting position and slightly leaning forward is sometimes helpful. In hospital or nursing home beds too often the patient is semisupine which is a difficult position to facilitate swallowing food. It is most important that members of the interdisciplinary team (speech therapist, nurses, occupational therapists) in collaboration with a radiologist ascertain the cause of the swallowing difficulty and institute measures to alleviate it.

The physical therapist assists with remobilization activities, range of motion exercises, strengthening of muscles, gait training, use of assistive devices and if indicated, the use of a wheelchair. Occupational therapists help with retraining activities of daily living, transfer skills, cooking, homemaking and use of self-help devices to facilitate acceptance of responsibility for self-care.

The speech pathologist helps the patient and family cope with communication problems. Both verbal and non-verbal mechanisms of communication are explored. The recreational therapist involves the patient in activities designed to improve social and physical skills and to alleviate feelings of loneliness and loss of confidence and helplessness. Social workers assess support systems, explore community resources, home health services and support that will keep the patient in a home environment. Management of urinary incontinence, prevention of pressure ulcers, constipation and other problems that afflict stroke patients are discussed in other chapters.

REFERENCES

1. Cutler, RW: Cerebrovascular Disease. Rubenstein, E and Federman, D (Eds.) in *Scientific American Med*, New York, 1982.

2. Sandok, BA; Furlan, AJ; Whisnant, JP. *et al.*: Guidelines for the management of transcient ischemic attacks. *Mayo Clin Proc, 53:*665, 1978.

3. Byer, JA; Easton, JD: Therapy of ischemic cerebrovascular disease. *Ann Intern Med, 93:*942, 1980.

4. Gresham, GE; Fitzpatrick, TE; Wolf, PA, *et al.*: Residual disability in survivors of stroke — the Framingham study. *N Eng J Med, 293:*954, 1975.

5. Garraway, WM; Whisnant, JP; Fulan, AJ, *et al.*: The declining incidence of stroke. *N Eng J. Med, 300:*449, 1979.

6. Editorial: Why Has Stroke Mortality Declined. *Lancet, 1:*1195, 1983.

7. Garraway, WM; Whisnant, JP; Drury, I: The changing pattern of survival following stroke. *Stroke, 14:*699, 1983.

8. Ruskin, AP: Understanding stroke and its rehabilitation, *Stroke, 14:* 438, 1983.

9. Hart, Geraldine: Strokes causing left vs right hemiplegia: Different effects and nursing implications. *Geriatr Nurs,   :*43, 1983.

10. Smith, DL; Akhtar, AJ; Garraway, WM: Proprioception and spatial neglect after stroke. *Age Aging, 12:*63, 1983.

11. Pedretti LW: *Occupational Therapy Practice Skills for Physical Dysfunction.* St. Louis: C.V. Mosby Co., pp. 276-295.

12. Geschwind, N: The apraxias: Neural mechanism of disorders of learned movement. *Am Scient, 63:*188, 1975.

13. Strub, RL; Black FW: *The Mental Status Examination in Neurology.* Philadelphia: F.A. Davis, 1977, pp. 85-106.

14.   Sacco, RL; Wolf, PA; Rannel, WB, *et al.*: Survival and recurrence following stroke: The Framingham study. *Stroke, 13:*290, 1982.

15. Schuchmann, JA: Stroke rehabilitation: Minimizing the functional deficits. *Postgrad Med, 74:*101, 1983.

CHAPTER 14

ARTHRITIS
(Snap, Crackle and Pop)

Old age is a time of heightened vulnerability to many disabling disorders including osteoarthritis, polymyalgia rheumatica and rheumatoid arthritis. Figure 14.1 shows the frequency of these disorders for each decade and especially indicates the increasing incidence of osteoarthritis and polymyalgia rheumatica in the frail elderly population.

Many patients have visible evidence of arthritis of the hands, knees and feet that are not incapacitating and require no therapy. Others may develop severe disabling joint disease that may restrict social activities and confine the afflicted frail person to the house, or room or cause them to be chairbound or bedridden. Loneliness and subsequently depression are predictable consequences of this

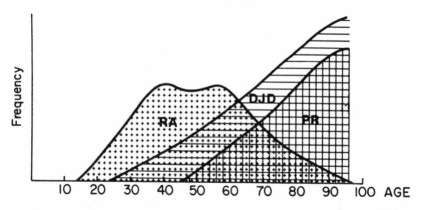

RA   Rheumatoid Arthritis
DJD Degenerative Joint Disease
PR   Polymyalgia Rheumatica

Figure 14.1. Frequency of arthritis with advancing age.

type of existence. Other consequences of arthritis in the frail elderly who already have some imbalance are falls, urinary and even fecal incontinence if unable to get to the bathroom or solicit help, constipation from lack of exercise and a sedentary lifestyle and pressure sores from immobility (Figure 14.2).

There are many effective treatments today to control symptoms of arthritis but there are few cures for chronic arthritic conditions of the elderly. This attracts many promoters of unproven cures, some of whom are sincere and well-meaning but misinformed believers, but also many who are disreputable profiteers. The claimed curative powers of moondust, copper bracelets, medical gadgets such as magnetic devices, certain vitamins, foods such as alfalfa tea, honey, vinegar, horse chestnuts and "immune milk" are unsubstantiated. Despite many books advocating special diets for the cure of arthritis there is no scientific evidence supporting these claims. Arthritis in the elderly requires early diagnosis, management of pain and inflammation, and relief of disability.

Rehabilitative measures should be practiced not only within the confines of a therapy department but also on the ward of a hospital, in the home and in the nursing home. Caregivers, whether

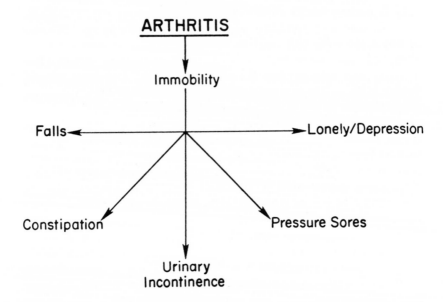

Figure 14.2. Consequences of arthritis.

they be nurses or spouse, should be instructed so that therapy can be continued at home or in the nursing home. Too frequently therapy is stopped after the patient goes home, only to be seen years later with severe disability that may have been prevented. Rehabilitative goals should focus on the ability of an arthritic patient to function in his environment. Measures should be instituted to improve muscular strength, range of motion, activities of self-care and mobility, but also modification of the environment to allow the patient to cope with their disabilities. Costs, psychological problems of the patient and the family, and nutrition are among other factors that affect outcome, the aggregate of which requires the services of an interdisciplinary team.

OSTEOARTHRITIS
(Degenerative Joint Disease, DJD)

Osteoarthritis, characterized by deterioration of joint cartilage and formation of new bone at joint surfaces, is the most common arthritic disorder. The incidence of the disease increases with age from 50% in the sixth decade to nearly 80% in the eighth decade. Radiographically, it is found in 40 million persons, yet only 5 million suffer significant symptomatology (2). The likelihood of pain and disability increases with advancing age. The role of physical "wear and tear" in the development of DJD is clear in advanced age involving primarily weight-bearing joints, but heredity and obesity may be possible factors. The aging process begins early in life in weight-bearing joints; visible signs appear on x-ray as early as the fourth decade of life.

DJD primarily involves areas of greatest stress such as the hands, knees, hips, cervical, and lumbar spine. Generally, the pattern of joint involvement in the hands identifies the type of arthritis. Bony swelling of the distal interphalangeal joints produce Heberden's nodes typical for DJD. Pain and stiffness lead to immobility which in some patients is severe enough to diminish capacity for self-care and may confine the patient to home, or require nursing home care. Neurological symptoms may occur with cervical spine arthritis.

The aim of treatment is to relieve pain and stiffness, to stop joint destruction and to enhance mobility. Diminished function from arthritis interferes with activities of daily living. The loss of hand, hip, and knee function interferes with independent living.

The fear of an impending permanent crippling disability is a major concern of anyone who develops arthritis. Asymptomatic patients can be treated by reassurance of the benign course of the arthritis, and even most patients with symptomatic arthritis can live active lives when managed properly, even though there is no cure for DJD. Ordinary daily physical activities do not sufficiently accelerate progression of the arthritis to force patients to develop a sedentary life (3). Management of arthritis is best accomplished with an interdisciplinary approach. Rehabilitation requires support of the physician, nurse, pharmacist, physical and occupational therapist. Drug therapy alone is not adequate and older people particularly require constant encouragement to stimulate them to continue the exercises needed to improve their range of motion and increase their strength.

Aspirin alone or combined with acetaminophen is effective in controlling pain. Non–steroidal antiinflammatory medications such as ibuprofen, naproxen, indomethacin, tolmetin, and piroxicam have been helpful. Occasionally, a corticosteroid injection into a joint (usually a knee joint) has relieved pain and allowed better mobility, but the number of repetitions should be strictly limited to no more than three per year and at intervals no less than every three months. Excessive activity on a weight–bearing joint brought about by pain relief after intraarticular injection of steroids may produce greater harm and becomes a major concern of this type of therapy. There is no place for systemic steroids in the treatment of DJD (3).

Physical and occupational therapy are important to strengthen muscles, increase range of motion, improve coordination, and to retrain older people to cope with activities of daily living. Application of heat, preferably moist, to relieve pain and stiffness can be safely accomplished with hot packs, warm baths, shower or whirlpool. Grab bars should be fitted in shower and bath areas for safety of frail elderly people. Heating pads and blankets should have safety features. Warm paraffin baths are helpful if carefully used to prevent burns. Simple measures often yield unexpected returns. Arthritis is often associated with weakness and atrophy of muscles that move the joint. Quadriceps muscle weakness associated with arthritis of the knee must be corrected to maintain joint stability and ability to stand and walk. A simple exercise to strengthen this muscle, recommended for an elderly patient sitting watching television commercials, is to extend the leg and hold it up against gravity until the commercial is over. This can be repeated with the opposite leg during the next commercial and alternated between each leg with subsequent commercials. Occupational therapists can teach alternative ways to accomplish activities of daily living, recommend simple devices with large handles for toothbrushes, eating utensils, and velcro strips in place of buttons. Canes, crutches, and walkers reduce stress on an afflicted hip or knee and enable frail elderly people with arthritis to increase mobility and walking distance. A cane should be properly fitted and held in the hand opposite the afflicted lower limb. Obese persons should lose weight.

Educational program for families given by members of the interdisciplinary team are important to ensure that therapy is conducted properly on the hospital ward and in the home. Therapy that occurs only during the short time that the patient is in the rehabilitation unit is not optimal. Patients require constant encouragement to continue exercise programs and health providers should be instructed by therapists to maintain an appropriate balance between rest and exercise whether in a hospital ward, nursing home, or at home.

Surgical treatment is beneficial for patients with intractable pain or disabling deformity. Total hip prosthesis has been remarkably successful in enabling older people to become more functional.

POLYMYALGIA RHEUMATICA

Polymyalgia rheumatica is almost exclusively a disease associated with the aged patient. It is almost never seen below age 50 and most patients are over 65 years old. It is more than twice as common in women and occurs universally in caucasians (3). This disorder is often misdiagnosed as fibrositis, degenerative joint disease, rheumatoid arthritis, bursitis or even attributed to psychological response to stress or tensions or a somatic complaint of depression. It characteristically consists of proximal muscle aching and stiffness in the pelvic and shoulder girdles. Stiffness is the major complaint, even more prominent than pain. Patients complain of difficulty getting out of bed or out of a chair because of stiffness. The onset may be gradual or the patient may progress overnight from a completely functional person to total disability. Fatigue, weight loss, fever and depression may be present.

On examination, the significant findings are limitation of motion and tenderness of muscles of involved areas. Muscular strength is surprisingly normal. The erythrocyte sedimentation rate is almost always elevated and is often a clue to the diagnosis (3, 4). Values are often over 100 mm/hr (Westergren Method) (3). Anemia may be present but the white blood count is normal. Muscle enzymes and biopsies are normal. Objective findings, therefore, are few and there is no specific confirmatory test for the diagnosis.

Response to low dose prednisone is rapid and dramatic in a day or two (3, 5). If no improvement results in a week the diagnosis should be questioned. Low dose prednisone may be required for months to two years in most patients (5), but others may need continued treatment. Aspirin or non-steroidal antiinflammatory drugs may provide relief but are usually not recommended to replace steroid therapy since they do not control the underlying arteritis.

GIANT CELL (TEMPORAL) ARTERITIS

Giant cell or temporal arteritis is closely related to polymyalgia rheumatica. Both may exist in the same patients. About 60% of patients with giant cell arteritis have symptoms of polymyalgia rheumatica before developing arteritis or during the course of the disease (6). Biopsies of temporal arteries show evidence of arteritis in 10 to 15% of patients with polymyalgia rheumatica who have no clinical evidence of arteritis (3). On the other hand, polymyalgia rheumatica may exist without ever developing evidence of arteritis.

Headache occurs in about two-thirds of afflicted patients typically localized to the temple. The artery may be swollen, tender, and nodular. Initially loss of vision may occur in one eye due to blockage in branches of the ophthalmic artery. Once established, blindness may be permanent. If the patient is untreated, loss of vision of the other eye may occur often within days or weeks (7). Most often, other eye problems precede blindness by several weeks or months. Pain in the jaw (claudication) with chewing due to inflammation of the facial artery occurs in approximately two-thirds of patients.

Fever, fatigue, weight loss, myalgias and arthralgia's such as found with polymyalgia rheumatica may occur. The patient may have scalp tenderness over the inflammed artery especially the temporal artery. An elevated erythrocyte sedimentation rate is almost always present. The diagnosis is confirmed by temporal artery biopsy.

Any person over 60 years of age who is diagnosed or suspected to have temporal arteritis must be started on high doses of prednisone to prevent visual loss (3, 7). Delay in therapy is dangerous and response to therapy is dramatic with clinical improvement within two to three days. Therapy must be continued for months with gradual lowering of the dose. The patient must be carefully observed for visual symptoms so that prednisone therapy can be reintroduced if relapse occurs.

RHEUMATOID ARTHRITIS

Rheumatoid arthritis can occur at any age (8) but its greatest prevalence is between the ages of 30 to 60 years. Many of these patients live to old age with evidence of arthritis or disability due to deformities and dysfunction but most often without active inflammatory disease. The onset of rheumatoid arthritis occurs in up to 15% after age 60 and clinical manifestations are no different than with younger patients in 75% of cases (5, 9). It involves the hands and wrists with typical metacarpophalangeal involvement in 60% of patients. The shoulder is particularly vulnerable being involved in 50% of older people. Morning stiffness and weakness of grip are characteristic findings with rheumatoid arthritis. In 25% of older patients, there is an atypical clinical picture with anemia, increased sedimentation rate and musculoskeletal manifestations that are difficult to distinguish from polymyalgia rheumatica, gout or pseudogout, or even an occult malignancy or infection (3, 9, 10).

Serological tests for rheumatoid factor are often positive with advancing age and may be misleading unless the titer is very high (10). Rheumatoid factor tests may be positive in 20% of people between ages 60 to 94 as an age-related phenomenon (11). This may lead to an erroneous diagnosis in an older patient with another form of arthritis.

Therapy for rheumatoid arthritis includes antiinflammatory drugs such as aspirin and other non-steroidal antiinflammatory drugs, physical and occupational therapy and in selected cases, surgery. Gold salts, antimalarial drugs, D-penicillamine, glucocorticoids and cytotoxic drugs (methotrexate, azathioprine, or cyclophosphamide) may be required if aspirin and non-steroidal antiinflammatory drugs are unsuccessful.

REFERENCES

1. Kaplan, PE: Rheumatoid arthritis and related diseases. In *The Practice of Rehabilitation Medicine*, Kaplan, PE and Materson, RS (Eds.). Springfield: Charles C. Thomas, Publ., 1982.

2. Scileppi, KP: Bone and Joint Disease in the Elderly. *Med Clin N Am*, 67:517, 1983.

3. Healey, LA: Rheumatology. In *Geriatric Medicine: Medical, Psychiatric and Pharmacological Topics*, Vol. I, Cassel, C and Walsh, J (Eds.). New York: Springer-Verlag, 1984, pp. 289-298.

4. Chuang, T; Hunder, GG; Ilstrup, DM, *et al.*: Polymyalgia Rheumatica: A 10-year Epidemiologic and Clinical Study. *Ann Int Med*, 97:672, 1982.

5. Giansiracusa, DF; Kantrowitz, FG: Rheumatic Disease. In *Health and Disease in Old Age*, Rowe, JW and Besdine, RW (Eds.). Boston, MA: Little, Brown & Co., 1982, p. 289.

6. Healey, LA; Wilske, KR: *The Systemic Manifestations of Temporal Arteritis*. New York: Grune and Stratton, 1978.

7. Goodman, BW: Temporal Arteritis. *Am J Med*, 67:839, 1979.

8. Brown, JW, Sones, DA: The Onset of Rheumatoid Arthritis in the Aged. *J Am Geriatr Soc*, 15:873, 1967.

9. Ehrlich, GE; Katz, WA: Rheumatoid arthritis in the aged. *Geriatric*, 25:103, 1970.

10. Ehrlich, GE: Rheumatoid Arthritis: It's Different in the Elderly. *Diagnosis*, 4:35, 1982.

11. Dequeher, DJ; Van Noyen, R; Vanderpitte, J: Age-related Rheumatoid Factors: Incidence and Characteristics. *Ann Rheum Dis*, 28:431, 1969.

CHAPTER 15

PARKINSON'S DISEASE

Parkinson's Disease is a chronic progressive degenerative nervous system disease. It is a leading cause of neurologic disability second only to stroke in patients over sixty years of age. Its greatest incidence is in the fifty to seventy year age group. The estimated prevalence is 100 to 150 per 100,000 (1). The clinical course is variable but the usual life expectancy from onset of disease is twenty-five years. In some, the course extends only a few to ten years. Therapy has reduced mortality and by increasing functional capacity has postponed the onset of crippling disability.

The primary lesion is a degenerative loss of nerve cells in the substantia nigra of the basal ganglia. The fundamental biochemical abnormality is a deficiency of the neuro-transmitter dopamine (1, 2, 3). The greater the loss of cells in the substantia nigra, the lower the concentration of dopamine. A deficiency of dopamine creates an imbalance of the striatal dopamine (dopaminergic) and acetylcholine (cholinergic) pathways with consequent enhancement of acetylcholine activity (2, 3). Normally the striatal tracts maintain a balance between dopaminergic (inhibitory) and its opposed cholinergic (excitatory) components. Any imbalance in these individual systems produces specific movement disorders. The theoretical goal of drug treatment, therefore, is to restore balance of striatal activity by reducing cholinergic activity with anticholinergic drugs and/or enhancing dopaminergic function with dopaminergic drugs (levodopa).

CLINICAL FEATURES

Characteristic clinical features readily diagnose this disorder. There are no laboratory or radiographic tests or procedures to identify the condition. The Parkinsonian syndrome consists of a classic triad of: Tremor, rigidity and bradykinesia.

Tremor is typically present at rest and usually involves the hand to forearm with rhythmic frequency of three to six cycles per second. It is present at rest and often disappears with purposeful movements. Tremor is ordinarily not present during sleep.

Rigidity is due to increased muscle tone producing resistance to passive motion. There is a "cogwheel" or "ratchet" resistance to passive movement of an extremity. This differs from spasticity. The patient sometimes complains of a feeling of stiffness.

Bradykinesia, a slowing of movement can be a most disabling feature of Parkinsonism. The patient appears to be immobile. There is a mask-like unblinking, fixed staring appearance and a paucity of facial expressions. Movement previously animated becomes deliberate and careful. Eating and dressing are painstakingly slow. Saliva accumulates in the mouth and throat as a result of diminished frequency of swallowing which may cause drooling at the lips. The voice becomes weak; there is reduced variability in pitch, stress and rhythm and sometimes, abnormal rates of speaking. The speech pattern may give the impression that the patient is depressed, demented, apathetic or unfeeling (4). Speech therapy may be helpful. Reading aloud from newspapers or magazines deliberately exaggerating each syllable with helpful criticism from family members makes it possible to improve speech so that it is understandable. Body posture is affected and the patient stands in a stooped, bent-over position. The head is bowed, the trunk is flexed forward, the arms are held close to the body, and in the standing position knees remain flexed (Figure 15.1). Because of the bent posture, the center of gravity is displaced forward and the patient takes short, rapid, shuffling steps which often progress into a festinating trot to maintain balance and avoid falling forward. The normal swinging of the arms is lost when walking. Leg lifting and swinging are virtually absent so that the patient is unable to flex the feet at the ankles, takes short, shuffling steps and often trips over scatter rugs, carpet edges, and other seemingly inconspicuous objects. There are greater problems with starting, stopping and turning. On changing direction, normally the head and eyes turn followed by the shoulders, trunk and legs. On the other hand, a Parkinsonian patient turns the entire body as if it were one unit. Rapid turns often produce loss of balance that may result in a fall. There is sometimes difficulty starting the process of walking so that the patient appears to be glued to the floor. Writing is abnormally slow with use of small letters (micrographia).

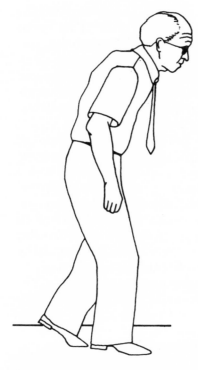

Infrequent blinking
Masklike facies

Arms adducted
→ ↓ Swing on walking
Trunk flexed forward
(bent posture)

Shuffling short steps
Festinating trot
Postural instability

Figure 15.1. Major clinical features of Parkinson's Disease. Adapted from Reference 2.

MANAGEMENT

Management is aimed at improving functional ability to permit patients to engage in normal or near normal activities. The family should be instructed in rehabilitative and supportive procedures and must monitor daily physical activities since it is largely in the home environment that these efforts will decide the rate of decline or retention of functional activity.

The patient must be attentive to all movement even those previously done automatically and must learn to perform activities, even walking, by thinking through each action. The patient must think about actions of eating, dressing, walking, turning and sitting (2). Distractions often impair functioning; patients may lose control, accelerate their gait, become unsteady and fall. There is difficulty in getting up from a sitting position especially from a low cushioned chair or davenport. A straight–back wood chair

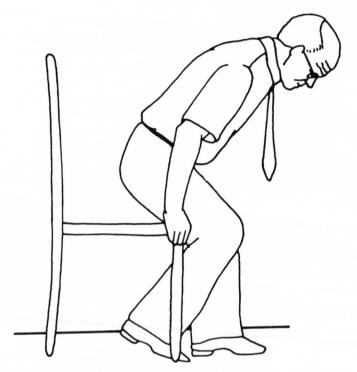

Figure 15.2. Rising from a sitting posture (see text). Adapted from Reference 2.

with arm rests is preferable (Figure 15.2). To stand up the patient must position the feet close to the chair with one foot under the chair, the other a half–step in front, slide forward to the edge of the chair, grab the sides of the chair or the arm rests with both hands, lean slightly forward or use a forward rocking motion while pushing with the hands (2, 5). Conversely, a common problem in sitting down is to fall into the chair which may result in sitting on one–half of the seat or falling. As with rising, concentration on each successive maneuver in sitting down requires practice. On approaching the chair, the patient carefully turns and positions the feet in a similar position as in rising and bends the trunk forward at the hips and slowly sits down using the arm rests, if present, for support.

Gait therapy must be continuously emphasized. The forward leaning and lack of associated arm movements cause instability, and inattention, even momentarily, may result in a fall. Walking can be improved by proper footwear and removing environmental impediments such as scatter rugs. In situations when the feet feel glued to the floor and the patient becomes immobile, a side to side rocking motion of the shoulders and body and deliberate swinging of the arms to simulate a walking motion is often helpful. Because of unsteadiness and a tendency to fall, the patient must be taught to walk around in a semicircle instead of turning abruptly (5). Building up the heels of the shoes may be helpful. Patients with Parkinsonism may have urinary incontinence for many of the same reasons that other patients have incontinence but additionally slow movement and rigidity may prevent quick access to the bathroom.

Modification of clothing and shoes improve daily tasks of dressing. Zippers, velco patches, snap buttons can replace ordinary buttons. Loafers or slip-on shoes are easier to manage than shoelaces. Canes and walking aids if needed must be carefully fitted for the individual patient. Range of motion and stretching exercises are necessary to prevent contractures especially when the magnitude of rigidity is greater with advanced disease.

The incidence of dementia in patients with Parkinson's Disease is much higher than in the general population (1, 6). By treating Parkinson's Disease and increasing mobility, other problems of caring for the patient surface. For example, wandering may be increased with betterment of mobility. Depression is also common in Parkinson's Disease for which both the patient and family will need therapy, education and guidance.

DRUG THERAPY

Mindful of the underlying biochemical imbalance, a decrease of dopamine associated with an enhanced acetylcholine activity, the logical therapeutic approach is to restore balance by replacing dopamine or reduce the influence of acetylcholine by using anticholinergic drugs (Figure 15.3) (1, 2, 3). Sometimes the judicious combination of both is effective. Levodopa is not initially indicated for early Parkinsonism but should be reserved for progressive functional impairment exemplified by difficulty in performing routine physical and social activities. It is effective therapy and allows the patient to continue normal activities of self-care for several years. Dopamine itself does not cross the blood-brain barrier, but levodopa (L-dopa) does and is, therefore, used for

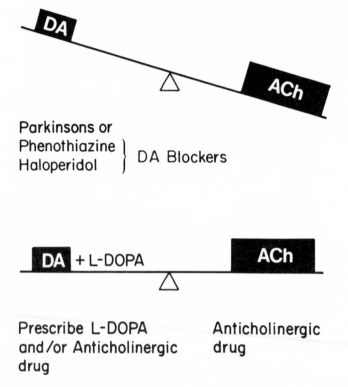

Figure 15.3. Acetylcholine (Ach)/Dopamine (DA) imbalance in Parkinsonism (top figure).
Balancing Ach/DA by increasing dopamine by adding L–Dopa or by reducing Ach by administering an anticholinergic drug (bottom figure).

therapy. Considerable levodopa is converted to dopamine by a decarboxylase enzyme in the body allowing only a relatively small amount of it to enter the brain.

> L–Dopa
> decarboxylase
> L–Dopa → Dopamine

Therefore, a decarboxylase inhibitor, carbidopa, is administered with levodopa (1, 2, 3). Carbidopa prevents conversion of levodopa to dopamine in the body allowing it to cross the blood brain barrier. Carbidopa itself does not pass the blood–brain barrier and, therefore, does not interfere with the metabolism of L–Dopa to dopamine in the brain. Available combinations are:

Sinemet 10/100 (ratio of 10 mg carbidopa to 100 mg levodopa)
Sinemet 25/100 (ratio of 25 mg carbidopa to 100 mg levodopa)
Sinemet 25/250 (ratio of 25 mg carbidopa to 250 mg levodopa)

Therapy is usually started with one tablet 10/100 Sinemet three times a day and slowly increased every two to three days to avoid nausea, vomiting and postural hypotension. If these side effects occur, switch to the 25/100 tablet to deliver more levodopa to the brain and reduce its peripheral body action. Despite its usual efficacy 20% of patients receive no benefit from Sinemet. Sinemet should be taken with meals to minimize gastrointestinal side effects.

Adverse reactions to levodopa are frequent, and careful titration of the dose is required to avoid them. Toxic delerium with confusion, an hallucinatory, angry, paranoid state, or postural hypotension may require discontinuation of the drug. However, a tolerance to this latter side effect usually develops. Abnormal involuntary movements of the mouth, tongue, and face produce involuntary grimaces, writhing or squirming of the body or restless legs, a clinical picture simulating tardive dyskinesia. A reduction of the dose may abolish this effect which sometimes unfortunately diminishes the effectiveness of the therapeutic response.

Amantadine, introduced for prophylaxis against Asian (A_2) influenza virus is transiently effective in treating Parkinsonism (3, 6). Its exact mode of action is unknown but it may enhance release of dopamine from dopaminergic neurons thereby making more available at the receptor site. It is slightly more effective than anticholinergic drugs but clearly less potent than levodopa.

Bromocriptine stimulates dopamine receptors and has been used as an adjunct to levodopa in patients whose response to the latter is decreasing (3).

Anticholinergic drugs have been used for many years to dampen cholinergic overactivity by blocking the action of acetylcholine. The effects are variable but clearly are not nearly as beneficial as levodopa. The major ones used are: trihexyphenidyl (Artane), benztropine mesylate (Cogentin), procyclidine, (Kemadrin), biperiden (Aikineton), cycrimine hcl (Pagitane Hcl).

Antihistamine drugs, diphenhydramine (Benadryl) 25–100 mg have anticholinergic properties and, therefore, have an effect on symptoms of Parkinsonism. Orphenadrine hydrochloride

(Disipal) and chlorophenoxamine (Phenoxene) are antihistamine drugs that have been used to treat this disorder.

The limiting factor in the use of anticholinergic and antihistsmine drugs are the undesirable side effects which are especially deleterious in older people. Blurred vision, dryness of the mouth, constipation, urinary hesitancy, retention or even overflow incontinence in patients with prostatic obstruction, tachycardia, drowsiness, confusion, hallucination and nightmares. The elderly are particularly prone to develop all of these side effects and are susceptible to developing severe mental disturbances. These symptoms disappear after the anticholinergic drug is either discontinued or the dose lowered. Anticholinergic drugs have a place in the treatment of Parkinsonism but must be carefully monitored in older people.

DRUG-INDUCED PARKINSONISM

Drugs are a frequent cause of Parkinsonism especially the antipsychotic (neuroleptic) drugs such as the phenothiazines and butyrophenones (haloperidol). These drugs block the dopamine receptors resulting in an increased acetylcholine synthesis and, therefore, cholinergic response, a situation similar to the dopamine-acetylcholine imbalance observed with idiopathic Parkinson's Disease. The onset of clinical symptoms occur soon after receiving these drugs and the symptoms remit after cessation of the drug or with the addition of an anticholinergic antiparkinsonism medication. Some antipsychotic drugs with anticholinergic action (thioridazine) when given in an appropriate dose sufficient to block the cholinergic response may control or diminish the Parkinsonism symptoms. Others without the pronounced anticholinergic effect (haloperidol) produce Parkinsonism more frequently. It has been recently observed that the prevalence of drug-induced cases is probably underestimated and that it can even occur with small doses of thioridazine previously considered a safe dose in elderly people (7). Drug-induced Parkinsonism should not be treated with L-dopa since the action of the antipsychotic drug works by blocking dopamine action.

TARDIVE DYSKINESIA

The late onset (tardive) of abnormal movements (dyskinesia)

is associated with long-term use of antipsychotic drugs such as phenothiazines and the butyrophenones (8, 9, 10). It is seen more frequently in the elderly especially in nursing homes and other long-term facilities because of the increasing use of antipsychotic drugs (9).

Hyperkinetic abnormal movements of the tongue, smacking of the lips, puckering, fly-catching motions, grimacing, and blinking are the buccal-facial-lingual components of this disorder. Older persons with poorly fitting dentures, however, may have some oral movements similar to tardive dyskinesia. Restless legs rocking or tapping of the toes or heels, patting the hands on the thighs are other features.

Patients are usually embarrassed by these movements, friends, relatives and onlookers may be annoyed and social activities are, therefore, restricted. It may cause inability to wear dentures, and makes eating and drinking difficult. Symptoms usually increase with anxiety or during times that a patient senses he/she is being observed, but abate during sleep.

Recovery occurs in about on-third of tardive dyskinesia patients within 6 months after antipsychotics are discontinued, others may improve gradually over 36 months, while a small percent are irreversible (11).

Other drugs known to produce tardive dyskinesia are L-dopa, amphetamines and reserpine (10).

BENIGN ESSENTIAL TREMOR

In older people, this disorder is frequently misdiagnosed as Parkinson's Disease. Lack of association with rigidity, bradykinesia or postural instability clearly separates the two disorders. Benign essential tremor is a postural tremor usually involving the upper extremities, head and neck rather than appearing at rest except when severe (12). It does not respond to antiparkinsonian medication. The tremor is frequently hereditary and often begins in early life but can occur at any age. If the tremor begins in old age it is referred to as senile tremor.

Essential tremor increases under emotional stress. Tremor of the hands increases when writing or bringing food or liquid to the mouth. It improves with rest, sedative drugs, alcohol and beta-adrenergic blockers such as propranolol, or nadolol.

REFERENCES

1. Yahn, MD: Early Recognition of Parkinson's Disease. *Hosp Pract*, p. 65, 1981.

2. Duvoisin, RC: *Parkinson's Disease: A Guide for Patient and Family.* New York: Raven, 1978.

3. Hoehn, MM: Recent Advances in the Treatment of Parkinsonism. *Drug Therapy (hospital)*, 7:81, 1982.

4. Scott, S; Caird, FI: Speech Therapy for Patients with Parkinson's Disease, *Br Med J, 283:*1088, 1981.

5. Aita, JF: Why Patients with Parkinson's Disease Fall. *JAMA, 247:*515, 1982.

6. Lieberman, AN: Treatment of Advanced Parkinson's Disease, *Geriatr Med Today,* 2:31, 1983.

7. Murdock, PS; Williamson, J: A Danger in Making the Diagnosis of Parkinson's Disease. *Lancet, 1:*1212, 1982.

8. Ehrensing, RH: Tardive Dyskinesia. *Arch Intern Med, 138:*1261, 1978.

9. Portnoi, VA; Johnson, JE: Tardive Dyskinesia. *Geriatr Nurs,* p. 38, 1982.

10. Anath, J: Tardive Dyskinesia: Myths and Realities. *Psychosomatics, 21:*389, 1980.

11. Berger, PA: Tardive Dyskinesia: Recent Developments. *Inter Drug Ther Newsl, 15:*17, 1980.

12. Truax, WD: Five Common Tremors: Classification, Key to Therapy. *Postgrad Med, 74:*68, 1983.

CHAPTER 16

DRUGS FOR OLDER PEOPLE

MEDICATION GUIDELINES

We live in a time when drugs are overvalued for their capability to provide a problem–free life. In every patient-doctor encounter, there is a tacit expectation that for every problem there is a medication. However, the judicious use of drugs in older people improves well–being and quality of life. Greater medication usage in the elderly is not altogether inappropriate since older people have one or more chronic diseases which may require medication for proper management. Appropriate medication should not be withheld because of old age. Nonetheless, the clinician must prescribe drugs sensibly and cautiously with the realization that every problem cannot be solved with a drug, that no drug will reverse the aging process, and adverse drug reactions are more common in the elderly.

Modern medicines are strikingly successful in the treatment of many disorders but it would be an unusual expectation to believe that the use of potent medications will selectively improve our quality of life without introducing problems. Therefore, along with the benefits of drugs come risks. The elderly have more illnesses, take more than 25% of prescription medications and have a higher incidence of side–effects than their younger counterparts (1). Those with multiple concurrent problems receive from three to twelve drugs per day excluding over-the-counter preparations (2). There is a two to seven–fold higher incidence of adverse drug reactions in the elderly (3, 4). The rate of adverse drug reaction progressively increases with each decade. Adverse drug effects are twice as common in the seventh and eighth decades compared to a 40 to 50 year old group (12 to 25% vs 7.5 to 12%) (1). About 5% of hospital admissions are due to adverse drug reactions (5), with a significantly greater number occurring in those over 70 years of age. Approximately three-fourths of drug reactions are predictable and preventable. A safe rule in prescribing for the elderly is to use the minimal number of drugs and the simplest regimen. Medication problems must be especially addressed in nursing homes whose residents have three or more concurrent problems and are receiving between four and seven different drugs each day (6). This frail elderly group with borderline physiological reserves are ingesting large doses of potent medications which cause problems often attributed to the dwindling effects of age. Inappropriate tranquilization unfortunately is a common practice in the nursing home setting.

PROBLEMS WITH COMPLIANCE

After undergoing expensive diagnostic studies it is assumed by health professionals that patients comply with their medication schedules. It is, therefore, surprising that almost 50% of patients take medication improperly (7). They may take none of their medications, prematurely discontinue a medication, take too little, take too much, take them at the wrong time, or use drugs not prescribed by the physician.

A recent example of "more is better" is an 80–year–old agitated patient who was treated at home with haldoperidol. The wife thought that if one tablet was good for her husband eight tablets a day would be that many times better to hasten control of agitation. The patient predictably not only became more docile but rigidity and immobility due to florid Parkinsonism ensued. Symptoms prevented the patient from getting to the bathroom and incontinence was the problem that resulted in hospital admission. After discontinuation of haldoperidol therapy several weeks elapsed before the patient recovered.

The consequences of non–adherence to a drug regimen are shown in Table 16.1. The futility, waste of time and resources are staggering. The patient not only does not benefit but health may even be jeopardized. Health care professionals must be alert to the recognition and correction of problems of drug compliance.

Patients do not adhere to a drug regimen for many reasons (Table 16.2). Certain chronic diseases that produce no or few symptoms such as hypertension are more often associated with nonadherence to a drug regimen (8). Conversely, medications used to relieve acute symptoms such as shortness of breath or edema in a patient with congestive heart failure are linked to com-

TABLE 16.1
CONSEQUENCES OF NONADHERENCE TO DRUG REGIMEN

- Untreated illness
- Wasted money for doctor, laboratory, x-ray studies
- Wasted money for unused medicine
- Wasted health care staff time
- Expense for assessment and treatment of adverse drug reactions

TABLE 16.2
MAJOR FACTORS IN NONADHERENCE TO DRUG REGIMEN

Type of Illness
- Chronic Disease
- Illness not perceived as serious
- Psychiatric and psychologic problems
    Dementia — forget to take medicine
    Anxiety and fear about illness
    Denial of illness or need for therapy
    Fear of dependence on medicine

Specific Disorders
- Poor vision — inability to read instructions
- Arthritis
- Neurologic disease } Unable to open pill bottle

Economic and Social Factors
- Cannot afford medication
- Decrease dose and frequency to save money
- No transportation to pharmacy
- Poor support system (family, etc.)

Drug Regimen Factors
- Regimen too complicated
- Multiple drugs (more than 3)
- Incompatable dosage schedules
- Verbal instructions only — failure to comprehend therapy
- Borrowing and lending medicines
- Using old medicines
- Self-medication — more is better
- Disagreeable taste
- Duplicate medications prescribed by different physicians
- Adverse or unpleasant drug reactions
- Feels better — discontinues medicine

pliance. However, even in these situations patients stop taking their medications as soon as symptoms disappear. Others stop medications before the drug has been taken long enough to be effective. Other obvious factors shown in Table 16.2 engender noncompliance. Efforts to remove factors associated with non-adherence to drug therapy should be a major concern of all health professionals (7, 8, 9). Compliance can be considerably improved by patient education which encompasses informing them about their illness, enlisting their acceptance of responsibility for following prescribed therapy, and providing written and verbal instructions. Printed drug information instructions are now available specifically for elderly patients for most drugs through the American Association of Retired Persons (AARP). People can accept responsibility for their own health care only if they are adequately informed by health professionals. How a patient uses the advice is dependent on the motivation of the patient and/or family.

DRUG EDUCATION FOR OLDER ADULTS

Members of the interdisciplinary team especially the physician, pharmacist and nurse have a responsibility to educate the patient and family about their drugs. The responsibility of the pharmacist on an interdisciplinary team is even more extensive including education of the health care team, the patient and the caregiver. The pharmacist's role is to:
1. Educate the professional staff about drugs in the elderly.
2. Review prescriptions or hospital order records for appropriate dose, drug reactions, or drug interactions.
3. Recommend more effective and less costly drugs.
4. Simplify drug regimens.
5. Educate patient and caregivers about drugs prescribed:
   a. verbal instructions
   b. written instruction (drug information pamphlets).

The nurse plays a central role in monitoring medications particularly in nursing homes. Residents are often given too many drugs, others may not receive their medications, the resident may not swallow the medication and spits it out when the nurse leaves. An indefensible practice in some nursing homes is the control of patients with drugs, a tendency to sedate or tranquilize the patients who become too active or independent and complain too much about the food and service, thereby disrupting regimented routines of an unsympathetic staff. The consequences of overuse of sedatives and tranquilizers are confusion, incontinence and falls, all of which are too frequently encountered in nursing homes where personnel fail to anticipate complications from drugs. This attitude and practice does not prevail in nursing homes with an informed enthusiastic nursing staff who are sensitive to patients' needs.

DRUG METABOLISM

Aging is associated with declining physiologic processes which affect the way that older people handle certain drugs as compared to their younger counterparts (1, 10). Changes in body composition such as a decreased muscle mass, increased fat and decreased water content within the body may influence drug distribution and produce an overdose in the elderly if given the same dose as prescribed for a younger person. The binding of drugs by plasma proteins is sometimes altered due to decreases in plasma albumin. Some decrease in albumin may be age-related but more significant changes occur with undernutrition or underlying disease. By decreasing protein binding of a drug, a greater amount of free drug is available at tissue receptor sites and consequently there is an increased risk of adverse side effects.

Drugs are removed from the body principally by two routes: 1) Metabolism in the liver to active metabolites or to inactive substances with subsequent excretion in the urine, and 2) elimination of unchanged drugs by the kidney (10). The kidney is the major organ for elimination of numerous drugs. Age-related loss of renal function is responsible for a reduced capacity to dispose of drugs or their metabolites. Renal blood flow and glomerular filtration rate decrease with the aging process. An approximately 50% reduction of glomerular filtration rate occurs between age 30 and 80 years. A serum creatinine level is traditionally used as a simple test to measure renal function. In the elderly, however, the results can be deceiving. Creatinine is produced in muscle and since muscle mass is reduced with age, an elderly person may have a normal serum creatinine level even if there is associated renal impairment. Therefore, the dosage of renally excreted drugs such as digoxin, or aminoglycoside antibiotics should never be based on a serum creatinine level but rather on creatinine clearance which is a measure of glomerular filtration rate. If this test is unavailable the health professional should assume that renal function is decreased by 50% and adjust the drug dosage accordingly.

Aging is associated with a decrease in liver size, hepatic blood flow and hepatic function. Undernutrition has been implicated in producing fewer enzymes or less enzyme activity and thereby reduction in drug metabolism. Generally hepatic blood flow is a major factor in liver clearance for drugs that are rapidly extracted by the liver such as propranolol and lidocaine. Since liver blood flow is reduced in the elderly there is a decrease in extraction and metabolism of these drugs and liver clearance is decreased. Reduced liver drug metabolism in the elderly occurs with antipyrine, prazepam, flurazepam and theophylline. Cigarette smoking increases microsomal liver enzymes in young adults and, therefore, hastens metabolism and excretion of drugs such as theophylline, diazepam (valium) and chlordiazopoxide (librium). In the elderly, however, cigarette smoking has a more limited capacity for inducing microsomal enzymes suggesting that the dose of theophylline should not be arbitrarily increased in elderly smokers (10). Clearly more experimental data on the complex interaction between the drug, environment and physiological changes in the elderly are needed to provide better guidelines for rational treatment with drugs.

SPECIFIC MEDICATIONS

A wide variety of adverse reactions occur with medications administered to the frail elderly. The frail elderly are particularly susceptible to the development of postural hypotension and confusion which have many consequences for this age group (Figure 16.1). Falls, myocardial infarction and cerebrovascular events occur more frequently from hypotension in the elderly . Drugs that have been implicated in causing postural hypotension and confusion are shown in Table 16.3.

Diuretics

Diuretics along with bed rest, salt restriction, and digitalis are the basic elements in the treatment of heart failure. Diuretics, commonly used for treatment of hypertension and congestive heart failure frequently produce adverse reactions in the elderly. The major problems complicating diuretic therapy are shown in

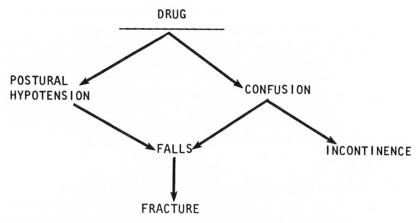

Figure 16.1 Major sequence of problems due to adverse reactions to drugs in the frail elderly.

TABLE 16.3 MAJOR DRUGS CAUSING:	
Postural Hypotention/Syncope	*Confusion*
Antidepressants { Tricyclics, Monamine oxidase inhibitors	Digoxin
	Cimetidine
	Dilantin
Antipsychotics (phenothiazines and butyrophenones)	Benzodiazepines Dalmane, Valium, etc.
Antihypertensives — Guanethidine Prazosin Methyldopa	Antidepressants
	Steroids
Diuretics	Barbiturates
Nitrates	Alcohol
Disopyramide (Norpace)	
Alcohol	
Levodopa	
Dipyridamole (Persantine)	

Figure 16.2. Diuretics eliminate the retention of salt and water, increase the rate of urine formation, and contract the body fluid volume. Some diuretics cause a significant urinary loss of potassium and produce hypokalemia (low plasma potassium), especially

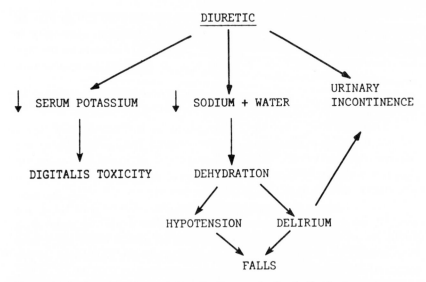

Figure 16.2. Complications of diuretic therapy in the frail elderly.

in an elderly person with an inadequate dietary potassium intake. Other factors that contribute to potassium deficiency are loss of appetite, vomiting and laxative abuse. A deficiency of potassium is particularly dangerous for the patient with congestive heart failure who is taking a digitalis medication. The administration of a diuretic that causes potassium loss to a patient who is on digitalis therapy often produces digitalis toxicity.

Older people are more prone to develop salt and water depletion (dehydration) with diuretic therapy. Postural hypotension and confusional states (delirium), therefore, may be consequences of diuretic therapy that may lead to falls. Diuretics may cause urinary incontinence during sleep in older people if a dose is administered too late in the evening. Another expected cause of incontinence occurs in an elderly male with prostatic hypertrophy who may develop overflow incontinence after receiving a diuretic. Older patients who develop dehydration may become confused (delirium) and become incontinent. A brisk diuresis may occur in a patient with limited mobility who may not be able to get to the bathroom in time.

Clinicians must anticipate complications due to durietic therapy in susceptable old people and monitor for deranged serum electrolytes and orthostatic blood pressures. Adverse reactions are frequent in the elderly and it behooves the health care team to be aware that edema which is so common in this frail group may be due to other causes such as venous insufficiency, especially in dependent extremities of sedentary people. Overvigorous therapy for the wrong diagnosis is more apt to lead to complications.

Digoxin

Digoxin is a commonly used drug in the elderly and toxic effects have been appearing with increasing frequency. There is a narrow dosage range between therapeutic efficacy and toxicity. Approximately 70% of digoxin is excreted by the kidneys. A reduction of digoxin excretion is commensurate with an age-related decline in glomerular filtration rate. Since less digoxin is cleared from plasma to be excreted into the urine the same dose given to an 80-year-old person results in about twice the blood concentration as compared to a young adult. Therefore, lower doses of digoxin should be used in the elderly.

Other factors that contribute to digitalis toxicity in the elderly are a low plasma potassium level (often related to diuretic treatment for heart failure), hypothyroidism, medication errors, and interactions with quinidine, verapamil, or nifedipine used to treat cardiac problems, but which cause a rise in serum digoxin levels (11, 12, 13). Digoxin doses should be reduced when these drugs are used concurrently.

Digoxin toxicity may cause loss of appetite, gastrointestinal discomfort, hazy vision, restlessness, weakness, fatigue, depression, bad dreams, delirium, and life threatening disturbances in heart rhythm (1, 14). Digitalis delirium is sometimes misdiagnosed as senile dementia. Any behavioral change or worsening of an underlying dementia in an elderly patient taking digitalis should alert the health care provider to the possibility of digitalis toxicity.

Digoxin is often prescribed for shortness of breath or swelling of lower legs which are clinical manifestations of heart failure. However, shortness of breath on exertion in a frail elderly person may be related to age-related diminished physiological reserves or lung disease such as emphysema and edema of the lower extremities is frequent in sedentary older people who have venous insufficicinecy. Digoxin is wrongly prescribed for many of these older people despite the lack of clinical benefit from its administration. The need for digoxin therapy should be reassessed in elderly patients who are in sinus rhythm with consideration for discontinuation of the medication for those in whom the reason for initiating therapy with the drug are inadequate (15). Withdrawal from digoxin should be carefully supervised. Digoxin should not be withdrawn from patients with atrial fibrillation or those with a history of rapid atrial arrhythmia.

ANTICHOLINERGIC EFFECTS

Anticholinergic drugs are used extensively in the elderly. Table 16.4 shows the major drugs that have anticholinergic effects. The concurrent use of several drugs is common and, therefore, the elderly are at high risk for developing anticholinergic side effects. Adverse side effects include dry mouth, constipation, blurred vision, tachycardia, hyperthermia, flushed faces, urinary retention, confusion, agitation, somnolence, visual hallucinations, picking at bedclothes, and sometimes coma. Older people without classical symptoms may be mistakenly treated for delirium, dementia, or psychosis. Overflow incontinence or worsening of urinary retention may be precipitated in elderly males with bladder outlet obstruction from prostatic enlargement. The simultaneous use of neuroleptics, tricyclic antidepressants, and antiparkinson drugs may produce toxic confusion. Constipation worsens and fecal impaction may ensue. Dry mouth from diminished salivary flow may cause decreased dietary intake. Hyperthermia and heat stroke or heat exhaustion may be induced by anticholinergic drugs.

Sleeping Pills

Preoccupation with sleeping problems increase with advancing years. Indeed, almost 40% of all sedative–hypnotic medications are prescribed for the elderly (16). The benzodiazepines are most frequently prescribed for sleep. Many old people underestimate the amount of sleep that they actually get and many complain of lack of sleep even when they have been observed to get adequate sleep. Young adults traditionally obtain about eight hours of sleep each day. However, the amount of sleep is extremely variable in healthy individuals and some active healthy individuals get only a few hours of sleep each night without harmful effects. Sleep patterns change with advancing age. Old people seem to require less sleep, obtaining 6 hours or less per night. This is partly because they are less active. Older people, troubled by less sleep, thinking it is unnatural, ask for sleeping pills. Often, a simple explanation

TABLE 16.4
MAJOR DRUGS WITH ANTICHOLINERGIC EFFECTS

Atropine, propantheline (Probanthine)

Antipsychotic (Phenothiazines)

Tricyclic antidepressants

Antiparkinson drugs

Antihistamines

Antiarrhythmics: Disopyramide (Norpace)

Benzodiazepines: Flurazepam (Dalmane),
Diazepam (Valium)

of the changing patterns with age, avoidance of tea, coffee or alcohol in the evening and moderate exercise during the day satisfies the patient. Most older people take daytime naps, but since they have not gone through the ritual of undressing and going to bed it is not perceived as sleep. This pattern is often found in nursing homes or long-term care facilities and the patient or staff insist on a sleeping pill so that their behavior will be synchronous with the night time pattern of others. If such a patient is disruptive to others at night, activities can be devised to keep the patient productive during daytime. Older people take a longer time to fall asleep, and some awaken early in the morning. Others fall asleep easily but awaken several times during the night.

Insomnia may be caused by pain, shortness of breath, itching of skin, getting up to urinate, or other medical problems. Older people are more sensitive to caffeine and drinking coffee at night may be responsible for poor sleep. Sleep disturbances are common with depression, anxiety and acute confusional state. Patients with senile dementia may wander at night. Therefore, proper diagnosis of these disorders with treatment aimed at management of the underlying problem will ordinarily help the patient. It is inappropriate to prescribe sedative-hypnotic drugs for sleep disturbances due to depression or arthritis. Using a sedative-hypnotic for sleep disturbances due to sleep apnea syndrome secondary to chronic obstructive pulmonary disease is hazardous and may even be lethal (16, 17).

Sleeping pills are usually effective for only a few weeks and are not designed for chronic use. Patients who have been taking sleeping pills should be withdrawn over a period of a few weeks to prevent anxiety, insomnia and unpleasant dreams that often occur with sudden discontinuation. Frail elderly people are particularly susceptible to developing adverse reactions with even low doses of sleeping pills. Central nervous system reactions should be more commonly anticipated in patients who have a decrease in mental agility and borderline cognitive function and the use of sedative hypnotic drugs should be discouraged. These drugs should be avoided in patients who have a substance-abuse problem or alcoholism. The elderly develop more central nervous system disturbances with flurazepam (Dalmane), a widely used drug for the treatment of insomnia, especially with 30 mg/day dose. However, even at 15 mg/day dose reactions can occur in this age group. Confusion, unsteadiness, falls, diminished coordination and daytime drowsiness are the major side effects that increase progressively with age.

Antihistamines have been used to overcome sleep disturbances and are the active ingredients in most over-the-counter sleep medicines. They are associated with a higher risk of delirium than are the benzodiazepines in the elderly (17). Diphenhydramine hydrochloride (Benadryl) has even infrequently produced confusion in frail elderly patients. A warm glass of milk or a glass of wine may enhance sleep in elderly people.

GENERAL MEASURES
TO IMPROVE DRUG THERAPY

• Explain disease(s) and medication(s)
• Provide written instructions when possible
• Minimize the number of drugs used — only prescribe drugs that are really needed
• Simplify dose regimens
• Use large print and simple directions on label
• Ask spouse, relative, community nurse to monitor drug therapy if indicated
• Review drug regimen frequently, including nonprescription drugs such as aspirin, anticholinergics, antihistamines, laxatives, etc.
• Discontinue unneeded drugs
• Discard old drugs
• Do not always blame patient for noncompliance, look for reason
• Individualize patient education, individualize drug therapy
• General rule — use lowest dose in the frail elderly and increase gradually; the normal adult dose is often an overdose

- Always think of a drug reaction as a cause of symptoms in the frail elderly
- Provide medication calendar and/or color coding on label for keeping track of different medicines
- Use cups, egg cartons, or commerical compartmental container system if indicated
- Ask patient to bring medicines periodically on office visits
- Ask to see medications on home visits
- Use all health care professionals to reinforce patient education (nurses, nurse practitioners, physicians assistant, pharmacists, social workers and dietitians)

REFERENCES

1. Vestal, RE: Drug Use in the Elderly. A Review of Problems and Special Considerations. *Drugs, 16:*358, 1978.

2. Lamy, PP: *Prescribing for the Elderly.* Littleton, Mass: PSG Publication Company, 1980.

3. Seidl, LG; Thornton, GF; Smith, JW, *et al.*: Studies on the Epidemiology of Adverse Reactions. III Reactions in Patients on a General Medical Service. *Bull Johns Hopkins Hosp, 119:*299, 1966.

4. Hurwitz, N: Predisposing Factors in Adverse Reactions to Drugs. *Br Med J, 1:*536, 1969.

5. Melmon, KL: Preventable Drug Reactions: Causes and Cures. *N Eng J Med, 284:*1361, 1974.

6. Ouslander, JG: Drug Therapy in the Elderly. *Am Intern Med, 95:*711, 1981.

7. Riegelman, RK: Potholes on the Road to Compliance. *Postgrad Med, 71:*205, 1982.

8. Anderson, RJ; Kirk, LM: Methods of Improving Patient Compliance in Chronic Disease States. *Arch Intern Med, 142:*1673, 1982.

9. Blackwell, B: The Drug Defaulter. *Clin Pharmacol Ther, 13:*841, 1972.

10. Greenblatt, DJ; Sellers, EM; Shader, RI: Drug Disposition in Old Age. *N Eng J Med, 306:*1081, 1982.

11. Leahey, EB; Reiffel, JA; Giardina, EGV, *et al.*: Effect of Quinidine and Other Antiarrhythmic Drugs on Serum Digoxin. *Ann Intern Med, 92:*605, 1980.

12. Leahey, EB: Digoxin-Quinidine Interaction: Current Status. Editorial, *Ann Intern Med, 193:*755, 1980.

13. Stults, BM: Digoxin Use in the Elderly. *J Am Geriatr Soc, 30:*158, 1982.

14. Coodley, EL; Rodriguez, J: The Pharmacokinetic Consultation Service: A New Approach to Digoxin Therapy. *Drug Ther, 8:*81, 1983.

15. Johnston, DG; McDevitt, DG: Is Maintenance Digoxin Necessary in Patients with Sinus Rhythm? *Lancet, 1:*567, 1979.

16. Solomon, F; White, CC; Parron, DL, *et al.*: Sleeping Pills, Insomnia and Medical Practice. *N Eng J Med, 300:*803, 1979.

17. Thompson, TL; Moran, MG; Nies, AS: Psychotropic Drug Use in the Elderly. *N Eng J Med, 308:*134, 1983.

INDEX

A

Activities of Daily Living (ADL), 14, 79-81
Age-related changes
    biologic changes, 9, 24-33
    psychologic changes, 33-39
Ageism, 18-20
Alcoholism, 56-58, 67, 129, 195
Alzheimer's Disease
    caregivers, 98-100
    diagnosis, 96, 97
    management, 97-100
    pathologic changes, 95
Anemia
    iron deficiency, 49
    folate deficiency, 47, 48
Anorexia, 43, 69
Anticholinergics, 198
Anticipatory Medicine, 12, 13, 41
Antidepressant drugs, 194, 195, 198, 199
Antidiuretic Hormone (ADH), 31
Antiparkinson drugs, 183-186
Antipsychotic drugs, 100, 186
Aphasia, 165
Appetite, 43, 44
Arteritis, giant cell (Temporal), 176, 177
Arthritis, 171-178
    osteoarthritis, 173-175
    rheumatoid, 177, 178
    polymyalgia rheumatica, 175, 176
Assessment
    financial, 71
    functional, 13, 14, 74-81
    home, 71
    neurological, 77
    nutritional, 71, 72
    physical examination, 72-77
    techniques for interview, 64-66
Attitudes of health care professionals, 6, 7,
    19, 21, 22, 63, 85
Atypical presentation of disease, 14-16, 68

B

Bedrest, hazards, 58, 59
Bedsores (*See* decubitus ulcers)
Bereavement, 38
Biology of aging, 24-33
    body composition, 24, 25
    bone mass, 146, 147
    brain changes, 29
    gait and postural changes, 129, 130
    muscle fibers, 25
    sensory changes, 27-29
    strature, posture, 25
Bromocriptine, 185

C

Calcium supplements, 151
Cancer, prevention, 59, 60, 76
    screening examination, 60
Cardiovascular
    changes with aging, 32
    effects of exercise, 32, 53, 59
    examination, 75, 76
Caregivers, 21, 66, 71, 85, 86, 89, 97-100,
    168, 175
Carotid sinus hypersensitivity, 132, 133
Cascade pattern of disease, 11-13
Catheters, urinary, 115-118
Cerebrovascular Accident (CVA), 160-170
    transient ischemic attacks, 160-162
Cervical Spondylosis, 134
Complications, 11, 12
Confusion, 14, 48, 94, 127, 198
Constipation, 69, 119-124
    causes, 119, 120
    management, 121-124
    symptoms, 120, 121

D

Deafness, 68
Death and dying, 38